Information in the Brain

Information in the Brain:
A Molecular Perspective

Ira B. Black

A Bradford Book
The MIT Press
Cambridge, Massachusetts
London, England

This book was set in Palatino by DEKR Corporation and printed and bound in the United States of America.

Library of Congress Cataloging-in-Publication Data

Black, Ira B.
    Information in the brain : a molecular perspective / Ira B. Black.
        p.   cm.
    "A Bradford book."
    Includes bibliographical references and index.
    ISBN 0-262-02321-0 (hc)
    1. Molecular neurobiology.   I. Title.
    [DNLM: 1. Brain—physiology.   2. Mental Processes—physiology.
    3. Molecular Biology.   4. Neurons—physiology.   5. Signal
    Transduction—physiology.   WL 300 B627i]
QP356.2B53   1991
612.8'2—dc20
DNLM/DLC
for Library of Congress   90-13591
                                                                      CIP

To Janet and Reed

Contents

Preface

An early interest in philosophy, psychology, or behavior frequently evolves into a fascination with the organ of origin, the brain. However, its complexity of physical design, its multifarious functions from perception to motor control to memory, and its multilevel organization from gene to molecule, cell, systems, and behavior encourage an intensely focused approach. That focus is abundantly rewarded. Disorientation is held at bay, and much is learned about a narrow area of neural function. In fact, focus is so inordinately successful that original motivations and perspectives may be easily, and imperceptibly, abandoned. The impenetrable big picture is sacrificed to the tractable experimental detail. This brief book represents one attempt to reconstruct the picture.

Where do we begin? It may be helpful to define a crisis in the brain and mind sciences to provide context and direction. Harshly stated, these fields have yet to fulfill the promise of forging a conceptual synthesis. The fields, and their component subfields, have failed to evolve a common framework indicating how brain state relates to mind state. No systematic mechanistic vocabulary, no general theory interrelates mind, brain, and behavior. Until this ambitious goal is achieved, neuroscience and psychology, brain science and behavior will not have begun to approach the central mandate in the study of mind. The fields will remain disarticulated and incomplete, lacking causal cohesion. Neuroscience will continue to define physical mechanisms without addressing the significant questions in psychology and cognition. The mind sciences, conversely, will continue in a mechanistically sterile fashion, lacking the physical equipment required to place the process of mind on a firm, physical footing.

What is it, then, that we seek? Simply stated, we seek to understand mentation and behavior in molecular biochemical terms and, conversely, understand biochemistry in behavioral terms.

Increasing attention nevertheless is being directed toward the big picture. Striking advances in brain science have prompted attempts to understand cognitive function in neurobiological terms. At this early stage, efforts have focused on well-defined characteristics of neural structure, such as gross anatomical pathways. Similarly, computational models of the brain have incorporated some features of neural microcircuitry. Remarkably, these initial approaches have captured a number of qualities exhibited by brain systems and by cognitive functions that the systems execute.

These tentative successes are all the more remarkable for having occurred in a virtual cell biological vacuum. Because the most prominent models fail to incorporate modern neural cellular and molecular biology, they are particularly impoverished compared to biologically based brain function. One goal of this book is to utilize a series of new and radical insights derived from neuroscience to develop a novel formulation of the physical basis of brain function and mind.

Recent molecular approaches have led to new views that require a reformulation of brain function: the neuron and the synapse are emerging as unexpectedly dynamic entities that change from millisecond to millisecond, simultaneously storing long-term information. These new observations have fundamentally expanded definitions of the flow of information in the nervous system. Indeed conceptions of the very nature of neural information are undergoing marked changes.

The new discoveries allow consideration of the biochemistry of information processing and storage in the nervous system. Some of the possible molecular and cellular bases of cognitive function are discussed in detail. I focus on molecules that serve as signals, communicating information among neurons. Mechanisms by which environmental (and internal) stimuli alter these molecules and their functions are described in detail. I indicate how these molecules receive, encode, store, and transmit information. Perhaps unexpectedly, these insights lead to a reformulation of the nature of higher function in the nervous system, of the mutability of neural structure, and of the relationship of brain and environment. Instead of viewing the nervous system as a static, passive structure upon which the environment acts, eliciting stereotyped responses, the view here is that the nervous system can be understood only as an organic part of the entire biologic world.

Briefly, certain types of molecules in the nervous system occupy a unique functional niche. These molecules subserve multiple functions simultaneously. It is well recognized that biochemical transformations are the substance of cellular function and mediate cell interactions in all tissues and organ systems. Particular subsets of molecules simultaneously serve as intermediates in cellular biochemistry, function as intercellular signals, and respond in characteristic modes to environmental stimuli. These critical molecules actually incorporate environmental information into the cell and nervous system. Consequently these molecules simultaneously function as biochemical intermediates and as symbols representing specific environmental conditions. This book is about the transduction processes through which environmental information is transformed into neural biochemical language.

The principle of multiple function implies that there is no clear distinction among the processes of cellular metabolism, intercellular communication, and symbolic function in the nervous system. Representation of information and communication are part of the functioning fabric of the nervous system. This view also serves to collapse a number of other traditional categorical distinctions. For example, the brain can no longer be regarded as the hardware underlying the separate software of the mind. Scrutiny will indicate that these categories are ill framed and that hardware and software are one in the nervous system. The implications of polyfunction are illustrated extensively in the course of this book.

The principle of polyfunction is complemented by the recently discovered co localization of neurotransmitters and growth factors in neurons. That is, a single nerve cell employs multiple chemical signals to communicate with other cells and with itself. Moreover, many of the co-localized signals are independently expressed, regulated, and used, depending on environmental stimuli. As a result, a population of neurons may use entirely different combinations of signals at different times, dictated by the environment. Thus, different signal molecules may encode different environmental data, leading to chemical coding. Within a single (neuroanatomical) pathway, chemical circuits form, dissolve, and reform, in response to environmental cues. Changing chemical pathways are thereby impressed on a substrate of relative gross anatomic stability. The remarkably rich potential for information processing conferred by symbolic function, polyfunction, and co-localization is explored in detail.

Although this preview has focused on symbolic function and used intercellular signals as exemplars, these particular molecules occupy a special position in the nervous system for an additional reason: they serve to communicate. And in the brain, which contains approximately 10^{15} specialized intercellular junctions, or synapses, devoted to signaling, it is apparent that communication is central to function. I suggest, then, that the biochemistry of symbolic function and communication is central to understanding brain function and mind function.

Certainly, it may be argued, symbolic and communicative functions exist at many other levels of organization of the nervous system. These functions must be evident at the cellular, systems, intersystems, behavioral, and psychologic levels. Of course, this is true. However, my strategy is to identify the simplest units of symbolic function and communication and attempt to identify underlying process and mechanism. An understanding at the relatively rudimentary, molecular level may provide insights applicable to levels of far greater complexity.

In fact, we examine the explicit claim that certain molecules constitute elementary units of cognitive function. Of course, these units are embedded in specific cells that comprise functioning neural systems. However, important characteristics of the behavior exhibited by any system are determined by operational rules governing behavior of comunicative molecular symbols.

Consideration of polyfunctional, symbolic molecules provides access to an additional central problem in brain sciences—that of multiple levels. The nervous system functions simultaneously on the genomic, molecular, cellular, systems, behavioral, mental, and environmental levels. How are these putative levels interrelated, if at all? Can we understand behavior in terms of cellular and molecular function? In fact, as I describe extensively, the symbolic molecules mediate communication among levels. Functioning as symbols in signal transduction processes that convert one form of information to another, these molecules integrate multiple (apparently distinct) levels of function. As an example, these molecules are vehicles through which environmental stimuli gain access to gene regulation. Consequently the environment indirectly regulates neural genes that contain the blueprint and operating principles of the brain.

In a system with a direct interface with the environment, it is not surprising that there is constant reciprocal interaction. In fact, behavior changes the molecular symbols on which behavior is based. This dynamic interaction leads to a system in which symbolic information is in constant flux. Dynamic interactions further blur conventional distinctions among internal and external worlds and among brain, behavior, and environment.

Brain and mind comprise a vast, integrated representational system that subserves such varied functions as sensation, motor behavior, cardiorespiratory control, learning, and memory. Our charge is to define the fundamental structural units of function upon which the operation of this representational system is based. The task of identifying functional structures in the nervous system is particularly difficult. Unlike other biologic organ systems, the brain stores information about the external and internal worlds. The cardiovascular system, on the other hand, is in the circulatory business, and this endeavor, in all its complexity, is not about something else. Processes that are uniquely neural, uniquely cognitive, and uniquely psychic concern the manipulation of symbols and symbol sets. This is the central fact of neural and mental life and the central clue to the brain-mind connection. We explore the rules governing the behavior of molecular symbols to begin understanding the characteristics of brain and mind function.

Of necessity, this inquiry demands discussion of processes in molecular biology, biochemistry, cell biology, systems function, neurology, psychology, and psychiatry. I try to avoid the confounding jargon that contributes to the inaccessibility of subspecialty areas, but sometimes clarity demands the use of specific notations. Consequently a glossary is included to encourage communication among fields. In addition, each chapter begins with a telegraphic, synoptic overview to provide orientation. Although the book hardly constitutes a molecular biology for psychologists or a psychiatry for biochemists, one of my goals is to contribute to interdisciplinary inquiry. If it identifies any common ground of shared concepts and interests, then accessibility beyond the parochial concerns of any single field will have been realized.

Acknowledgments

The idea for this book arose from the communal source of the vast majority of ideas in the scientific endeavor: discussions with colleagues, teachers, and students. Most of these colleagues had little indication that their insights would craft a book and undoubtedly will be surprised to find their names cited here. A number of individuals have been particularly influential, generously sharing emancipating visions and unconventional views.

Mike Gazzaniga, a long-term friend and colleague at Cornell University Medical College, has ceaselessly labored toward the emergence of a truly interdisciplinary cognitive neuroscience. His endless stream of ideas, his constant intellectual challenges, and his unfailing, optimistic encouragement have been seminal. Mike seemed to engage me in a single ongoing dialogue that began at Cornell, extended to airplane and airport, continued at conferences in London, Paris, and Venice, invaded the international computer networks, resumed at Dartmouth, and continues unabated by telephone. The message has been loud and clear: if we are to craft a unified science, we must move beyond the safe, parochial confines of our comfortable subspecialties to an insecure no-man's-land of synthesis. The psychological risks far outweigh the intellectual, but the rewards are the very substance of the enterprise. This book is a modest step in that direction.

Leon Festinger was an inspired teacher and colleague who is now painfully missed. His contributions to this effort were enormous. Leon's severe intellectual standards, uncompromising criticism of imperfect concepts, and thorough disdain for triviality bore constant testimony to the inadequacy of preliminary drafts. His sense of humor, his sympathetic encouragement, and his knowledge of the nature of the struggle were a source of immense encouragement.

The members and guests of the McDonnell Foundation Panel on Memory unwittingly provided invaluable insights concerning the prototypical problem of memory from divergent viewpoints. Gary Lynch cogently argued for neurobiological mechanism in the hippocampus;

Bill Hirst demanded that biological explanation satisfy the psychological feat; Richard Andersen forged new ground, formulating a computational approach to experience-driven neuron ensemble formation in primate brain; Gordon Shepherd outlined a model for the dendritic integration of information at the cortical synapse; Richard Thompson elegantly described the roles of brain stem and cerebellum in mnemonic phenomena, thereby illustrating the distributed nature of information in the brain; Dave Premack patiently explained the role of pedagogy in primate behavior and evolution, providing a unique perspective. John Bruer of the McDonnell Foundation supported the entire undertaking with protective enthusiasm.

Jim Watson of the Cold Spring Harbor Laboratories provided a fertile home for the annual summer course on the Molecular Neurobiology of Human Disease that I helped direct with Xandra Breakefield and Jim Gusella. As always, I learned far more than the students. I am especially grateful to several individuals who generously taught us all with patience and with discussions that frequently extended to the early morning hours. Mort Mishkin treated us to a magnificent, evolving saga of the elucidation of cognitive systems in the primate brain. He entertained my most naive questions and explained with excitement and enthusiasm. He continually encouraged efforts to synthesize the molar and the molecular. Lars Olson continued to illustrate how the brilliant experimentalist can disarm the most formidable problems in brain science. Al Aguayo always found time to teach us that our most pessimistic views that brain neurons cannot regenerate are wrong. Marc Raichle modestly introduced us to the use of the new brain imaging technologies in novel approaches to the most baffling questions in cognition. Ed Herbert guided us through the world of polyproteins and their genes with gentle rigor. And Carlton Gajdusek expounded on slow viruses, stone age culture, cannabalism, physical anthropology, neurology, pediatrics, linguistics of the South Fore in New Guinea, and Western history in scintillating, marathon discussions from sunset to sunrise.

A number of colleagues in addition to Gazzaniga and Festinger reviewed incarnations of the manuscript. Fred Gage read an entire draft and provided critical insights, suggestions, and overview. Bob Hamill, a true physician-scientist, offered advice and perspective that improved the effort immeasurably. Bruce McEwen took the time to recommend important organizational changes.

I owe a special debt to scientific colleagues with whom I have shared laboratories; they have shared views, introduced me to new areas, and tolerated all my questions. Julie Axelrod at the National Institutes of Health touched a generation of scientists with his magic, intuition, and boundless excitement. Perry Molinoff taught that no experiment is too large or complex in the quest for answers or new questions. His optimism lies at the heart of the scientific search. Leslie Iversen guided me through Trinity College, Cambridge, and helped me embark on several rewarding scientific journeys. My colleagues in the Laboratory of Developmental Neurology at Cornell—Josh Adler, Manny DiCicco-Bloom, Cheryl Dreyfus, and Kuo Wu—have cheerfully withstood the endless speculations and abortive ideas. Elise Grossman, my colleague and friend, constantly encouraged and advised, frequently reading passages for comprehensibility. Her judgment has always been impeccable. Bettye Mayer contributed in many ways—at computer, library, and telephone. A group of gifted, generous graduate students provided a steady stream of scientific papers, slowing intellectual ossification.

Our work has received the unflagging support of a number of agencies and foundations that underlie the biomedical research effort in the United States. The National Institute of Neurological Disease and Stroke (NINDS) and the National Institute of Child Health and Development (NICHD) have been unwavering. Gene Streicher at NINDS and Gilman Grave at NICHD have always been available for advice and guidance. The National Foundation–March of Dimes has been a partner in these investigations, and special gratitude is expressed to Sam Ajl for his interest and support. The McKnight Foundation has allowed us to explore a number of novel avenues and has encouraged departures from orthodoxy. Their long-term support is a model for the entire scientific enterprise. The Familial Dysautonomia Foundation offered ongoing resources to study development of the nervous system. Bristol-Myers Squibb initiated a new program of unrestricted grant awards that allowed us to venture into new areas, driven primarily by curiosity and possibility; the neuroscientific community owes a great debt to the vision of Davis Temple, Bill Komer, and Tom McCann. The Juvenile Diabetes Foundation exhibited notable breadth and understanding in extending their reach to seemingly distant arenas to solve neurological problems of the diabetic—testimony to the forward thinking of Kenneth Farber and his associates. The Nathan Cummings family endowed a chair of neurology at Cornell, thereby contributing to the continued freedom of academia. Their thoughtful interest has been a source of encouragement.

Finally, I thank my wife, Janet, and son, Reed. Janet read many sections and offered gentle suggestions, a nearly impossible task for a fiction writer who lives the language. Reed, at eleven, exhibits the joyful curiosity and fearlessness that generates a new theory each day. He is a worthy guardian of the enthusiasm.

Introduction: Problems and Questions

A 72-year-old retired professor of English is felled by a stroke and enters the hospital unable to read but able to write spontaneously or from dictation. A totally blind patient is able to react appropriately to visual threat—a fist directed toward his nose. A man with Parkinson's disease, paralyzed and bedridden for five years, runs out of a burning nursing home and then collapses once again, immobile, on the front lawn. Damage to an area of the right (nondominant) parietal lobe reproducibly results in neglect of the left side of space, including the left side of the body, inability to dress oneself, and denial of all disease. An elderly woman with cardiovascular disease repeatedly bursts into crying spells but denies on questioning that anything is wrong. These well-documented clinical syndromes, almost regarded as routine by neurologists, psychiatrists, and psychologists, define some of the central mysteries of brain function.

Can we begin to understand these seemingly paradoxical disorders, and underlying normal functions, in biological terms? Do molecular, cellular, and systems bases of brain function explain these baffling cases? Where might an inquiry begin?

Chapter 1

A General Introduction to Communicative

Symbols

Functionalism—The Computer Metaphor—Hardware and Software—
Instruction and Selection—Structure and Function—Communication,
Growth, and Architecture—Connectionist Program—Reductionism—
Structure and Function in the Nervous System—Combinatorics—
Aboutness—Electrochemical Coding—Temporal Amplification—Molecular
Structure and Modularity—Mental Function and Cell Biology

The brain and mind sciences stand on an exciting threshold, analogous, perhaps to that occupied by physics at the turn of the century.
Neurology and psychiatry, experimental psychology and neuroscience, and ethology and sociobiology have yielded unprecedented
insights into brain function. Nevertheless, these fields have yet to
approach any plausible unifying concepts that begin to explain the
function of brain and mind.

One goal of this book is to indicate how the functioning cognitive
system is actually instantiated in the physical nervous system. I explore some of the rules of operation of the nervous system that are
responsible for cognitive and psychologic traits, characteristics, and
function. My goal, in brief, is to indicate that mind is a biologic entity.
One of our chores will be to understand how the laws and constraints
of biology endow the mind with unique qualities. In fact, I fully intend
to show that mental function cannot be adequately understood without detailed consideration of biologic mechanism and process. This is
not a claim that can be accepted out of hand. Let us consider the
alternatives.

The Functionalist Paradigm

The biologic view cannot be considered a majority opinion among
cognitive psychologists and philosophers concerned with mind. The
functionalist stance probably comes closer to representing the domi-

nant paradigm (for reviews, see Flanagan 1984; Churchland 1986; Changeux 1985). According to this argument, mental states are functional states that can be instantiated in a variety of physical substrata. In fact, a virtually infinite variety of physical systems may be capable of giving rise to the system we call mind. Consequently the proper sphere of endeavor for those interested in mind is psychology—not neuroscience, not neurology, and not biology. Moreover, the study of mind lives in cognitive psychology, computational psychology, and artificial intelligence. Mind is not to be understood in terms of brain science, which is merely one instance of implementation. Instead it can be studied and understood without recourse to associated or underlying hardware. Psychology, in the broadest sense, will uncover the rules, relations, and laws that govern mind function, and these will help in the evolution of a complete theory of mind. In contrast, study of the nervous system is an entirely different pursuit and in any case will not shed light on the mind. An understanding of neuronal function, synaptic communication, the operation of neural systems, and brain physiology will reveal only low-level nuts, bolts, and microchip details of little relevance to mind function. Elucidation of molecular function explains little about how cars run, televisions work, or computers operate. Nor should we confuse mechanics, carpentry, and plumbing with architecture and sculpture. Every field, every age has its reigning metaphor, and cognitive functionalism in the late twentieth century has the computer.

Baldly stated, computer hardware is to brain as software is to mind. The brain may house the circuitry, the chips, and the boards, but it is the program, the software, that is of interest if we want to decipher the strings of the mind. A program can be run on many different computers with diverse architectures. The electronic wiring diagram is of little relevance to understanding the nature of the program itself. The logic of the program, the logic of the mind is to be comprehended in the rules governing programming. Screwdrivers, pliers, and soldering irons are inadequate tools for decoding the logic of formal programs. The physics of vacuum tubes, transistors, and microchips reveals little about programs and the output they engender. Neurons, synapses, and neural systems reveal little of the mind, a functional program. So runs the functionalist view and the computer metaphor, stated in extreme terms to drive home the point.

Functionalist Fallacy and Muddled Metaphor

The evidence that I present and the view that I will develop in the course of this book represent a frontal assault on the functionalist position and the popular computer metaphor. Shorn of all detail, the software-hardware dichotomy is artificial. As we shall see, software and hardware are one in the same in the nervous system. To the degree that these terms have any meaning in the nervous system, software changes the hardware upon which the software is based. For example, experience changes the structure of neurons, changes the signals that neurons send, changes the circuitry of the brain, and thereby changes output and any analogue of neural software. In fact, mutability, flexibility, at many levels and in many domains, represents a central property of the nervous system. Extensive evidence indicates that the brain is not an immutable series of circuits of invariant elements; rather it is in constant structural and functional flux. The digital computer analogy is fatally misleading.

Experiential input changes the neurotransmitter signals that neurons send, changes the nature and number of synapses, changes the structure of neurons, changes the wiring of circuits. Since no one, to my knowledge, argues that mind does **not** happen to be instantiated in brain, the biologic dynamics can hardly be irrelevant. In fact, I shall develop the view, based on increasing evidence, that the properties we provisionally call mind are part and parcel of the nervous system, not a disembodied abstract. My task is to describe in detail how the function of the foregoing neural elements constrains, characterizes, and in the last analysis is mind.

This is a particularly optimistic view, suggesting that the study of mind does not violate all we have learned about the relation of structure and function in biology. Indeed, one compelling reason for regarding the functionalist paradigm with skepticism is that it is contradicted by a wealth of evidence in science in general and in biology in particular. For example, cognition may be regarded as a function of brain just as circulatory regulation is a function of the cardiovascular system. Blood pressure, heart rate, and peripheral perfusion arise from cardiac dynamics and arteriolar constriction, which, in turn are influenced by hormonal status, neural innervation, state of hydration, and other variables. The relationships are profoundly complicated and interesting but not mysterious, magical, or privileged. We need not step outside the cardiovascular system to understand the circulation. In fact, to do so involves great scientific peril. The cardiovascular system could simply be viewed as a fancy bit of plumbing, easily modeled with some tubing, a few check-valves, a diaphragm or two, several reservoirs, and a pump. Our contraption would capture some aspects of cardiovascular function, but it would not necessarily predict that the pump itself elaborates diffusible stuff that regulates circulation. It would not predict that many of the perfused gadgets or organs also release substances that communicate with the central pump, altering its function, and also talk to the nerves governing pump and tubing function. Such specific insights must derive from study of the cardiovascular system itself.

While selected aspects of cardiovascular function might be characterized by studying models, much of the richness of the principles governing function would be lost. Although it is reasonable, in principle, to assume that cardiovascular function could, in some crude fashion, be instantiated in a variety of artificial contraptions, study of these rough functional replicas cannot be regarded as a substitute for study of the real thing. The plumbing system we construct, however elegant, need imply nothing about neurotransmitters, hormones, receptor kinetics, receptor transduction mechanisms, depolarization-contraction coupling in vascular smooth muscle, water and salt balance, acid-base balance, and a myriad of additional mechanisms. Yet consideration of the cardiovascular system in the absence of these regulatory controls is incomplete. We will be discussing plumbing, not cardiovascular dynamics.

Entirely analogous arguments can be applied to every other organ system in the body. Renal dialysis units, prosthetic limbs, and hearing aids abound in many forms, yet none of the artificial devices captures complete functions of the appropriate biologic system. What evidence supports the contention that the mind occupies an entirely anomalous position in all of biology? There seems to be no precedent for the functionalist claim. Moreover, as we proceed, we shall see that there is a large body of contradictory evidence. Even with the rudimentary data available, the functionalist stance and the computer metaphor appear to be misconceived.

Relationship of Hypothetical Hardware and Software

By examining the relationship of presumed hardware and software in the nervous system, we may appreciate the difficulty of this approach in biology and simultaneously identify a number of central questions. As a first approximation, we can regard the structure of the nervous system, from neural subsystems to molecules, as "hardware." More specifically, hardware may consist of neural genes, molecular signals of communication, the physical apparatus (synapse) through which communication occurs, individual neurons, populations of neurons, and neuron systems. However, this micro and macro architecture also contains the algorithms, the rules of operation, the programs. As we shall see, the rules of operation are incorporated by the elements constituting organization at each level.

The characteristics of the program run by any subsystem consist precisely of the characteristics of the neurotransmitter signals used, the transmitter receptors expressed, the membrane ion channels activated and inhibited, the intracellular biochemical mechanisms employed, and the synapses activated, for example. These elements, among others, sum to give the program its frequencies, temporal pattern, and amplitude. The neuroanatomical organization of the system determines the readout, whether visual, visceral regulation, or motor. The software is not a disembodied entity, separate and distinct from the biology. The algorithms are composed of the rules of molecular biology, biochemistry, electrochemistry, and connectivity. There is no separate existence of a program, of a vitalistic homunculus. Where would the software, standing outside biology, come from?

One provisional answer might be the environment. The program may be transferred to the internal nervous system by the external environment. However, this constitutes a misreading of the relationship of environment and biology. Environmental stimuli serve to trigger biological mechanisms already present in the nervous system, thereby altering neural structure and function. The external world does not dictate the rules of neural function in an ongoing manner. Rather, the environment uses and chooses among the biological mechanisms that are present. The transduction process, which converts environmental stimuli into neural information, should not be mistaken for transfer of a program from external to internal world. The biological transduction mechanisms are preexistent in the nervous system and operate according to the rules of cell biology and biochemistry. The transduction process itself is part of the "hardware" of the nervous system. Simultaneously, however, transduction is "software." In fact, the molecules, the transformations of biochemistry, and the principles obeyed are both hardware and software. These terms, however, fail to capture the nature of neurologic function.

The environment does not "program" the nervous system. Rather, increasing evidence indicates that the environment selects among potentials for characteristics and processes already present in the system, thereby eliciting change. Mutability of the nervous system is not conferred by the environment; the external world triggers the potential for change that is already built into the system (for extensive discussion, see Piattelli-Palmarini 1979).

To use a rough analogy, programs are instructionist, but the environment elicits neural change through selectionistic mechanisms. Although the issue of selection versus instruction (nature versus nurture and the innateness controversy) derives from other areas of biology, it may shed some light on misconceptions in neurobiology. In partic-

[handwritten marginalia: "→ reminder one of Platonic archetypes!"]

[handwritten marginalia in left margin: "selectionist view"]

ular, consideration of this issue helps to emphasize the inadequacy of any presumed hardware-software divide in neural function.

It may be helpful to epitomize a selectionist view since it redirects attention away from the computer metaphor and defines the appropriate sphere of this inquiry. In brief, the extreme position holds that nothing is ever truly "learned," in the sense of isomorphic, de novo transfer of program from environment to brain. The environment simply triggers (uses, chooses among, fixes, combines) innate mechanisms and processes that already exist on the basis of biology. In Fodor's terms, this accounts for the apparent arbitrariness of environmental triggering stimulus with respect to behavior or "concept" triggered and the lack of "logical" relation between the two (Fodor 1979; Fodor and Pylyshyn 1988). An example from ethology is illuminating. Ducklings imprint on any moving object, treating it as mother; in other words, movement signifies mother. Fodor argues persuasively that this phenomenon is most readily understood in Darwinian (1859) terms, not in terms of concept learning. Stimulus movement does not confirm an avian hypothesis about the structure of motherhood; it does not transfer the mother program to the brain. The selectionist view, based on preexistent biological mechanism, allows for any degree of apparent arbitrariness. The relation between stimulus and response is evolutionary and may be logically arbitrary in terms of any discernible, ongoing exigencies. It most certainly is not a software-hardware relation.

The selectionist view also accounts for the relatively invariant nature of responses across members of a species to an environment that presents markedly different stimuli. If different environmental stimuli simply downloaded different programs, the radically different histories of individuals might be expected to result in grossly divergent behaviors, thought patterns, and emotions. But the behavior or emotion is not programmed by the environment; it is intrinsic to the nervous system. The environment simply releases the information already present in the organism, and that information is not usefully defined as either hardware or software. It is biologic information that must be understood in biologic terms, according to the rules of biology, not the rules of computers. Germane scientific questions may be physiological or evolutionary, but they certainly are not about semiconductors or computer programs.

On the other hand, it is the state of the world that determines which biologic mechanisms and processes are triggered and expressed. Nevertheless, the critical interaction is that of the external world with the innate biological system. Consequently we may most fruitfully focus on the biology itself rather than on chimeric concepts of software and hardware. In fact, altered architecture of the nervous system is one of the most important classes of mechanism generating altered function, quite unlike a simple software change. A significant portion of this book is devoted to examining the rules governing these changes, since altered architecture alters neural function and since these biologic changes are fundamentally different in kind from accustomed computer software changes. A brief preview of neural dynamics may add further perspective, before plunging into detail, and further distinguish the new view from the functionalist position.

Structure and Function: Dynamics of Neural Architecture

The architecture of the nervous system is subject to change at multiple levels of organization and in multiple domains. Altered architecture is associated with altered modes of processing and altered neural function. Description of changes in general terms may indicate how biology and silicon-based technology differ and may provide orientation. For the purposes of discussion, the organization of neural "hardware" can be divided into genomic, molecular, synaptic, cellular, and systems domains that underlie and generate behavior and mental function.

Emerging evidence indicates that the nervous system processes information by altering structure and function at each of these levels. The readout of specific genes is constantly changing, leading to the elaboration of different products central to information flow in the nervous system. For example, genes that encode transmitter molecules, which act as agents of communication among neurons, are subject to complex regulation by the environment (Black et al. 1987). Variable and differential expression of these genes leads to continuous change in the transmitters synthesized by any single neuron. Since multiple, different transmitters are co-localized to single neurons, remarkable combinatorial flexibility is realized. This represents one mechanism by which the molecular structure, the "hardware," of neurons changes over time, altering function. In turn, change in neurotransmitter expression and metabolism results in altered behavior and mentation, as I describe extensively in subsequent chapters. Thus, a basic change in hardware leads to change in behavioral readout.

The structure of the synaptic apparatus, the communicative junction between neurons, also changes in response to environmental stimuli. Experience changes the molecular structure of the synapse (Wu and Black 1989; Bailey 1989), the morphology of the synapse, and even the number of synapses (Greenough 1984), leading to altered efficiency of communication and altered behavior. These structural changes in neural communicative connectivity occur at the heart of a system that functions through communication. This is hardly a change of "software."

The foregoing changes alter the neuroanatomical and neurochemical organization of neural subsystems, changing behavioral output of the nervous system. It should be apparent that function of the nervous system cannot be considered in the absence of knowledge of the rules of structural change, the rules of biology. Neural function derives from these rules, indeed, is a manifestation of these rules. There is no separate program, no separate software beyond the rules of biology that govern neural function.

Communication, Growth, and Altered Architecture: Emerging Unity

Increasing evidence indicates that ongoing function, that is, communication itself, alters the structure of the nervous system. In turn, altered structure changes ongoing function, which continues to alter structure. The essential unity of structure and function is a major theme of this book and is discussed extensively. Several general examples may further illuminate the inadequacy of the software-hardware construct and the hardwired computer metaphor.

In one example, coincident electrical activation of different incoming neural pathways to the same nerve processes leads to a strengthening of synapses in the rat hippocampus, the part of the brain that appears to be critical for spatial memory. Synaptic strengthening in this instance has been termed long-term potentiation (LTP), and has attracted particular interest since it might be associated with memory mechanisms (Bliss and Lomo 1973; Andersen et al. 1980; Lynch 1986). This process is especially relevant to this discussion because it involves alteration of synaptic structure. Evidence suggests that LTP is associated with an increase in the number of synapses and with changed structure of individual synapses (for review, see Lynch 1986). In fact, a particular excitatory neurotransmitter, glutamate, appears to elicit these changes by interacting with specific receptors on hippocampal neurons (for review, see Nicoll 1988; Nicoll et al. 1988). In summary, a transmitter signal, which is known to convey millisecond-to-millisecond excitatory information, also regulates circuit architecture by stimulating synaptic growth. In this system, then, signal communication, growth, altered architecture, altered neural function, and memory are causally interrelated; there is no easy divide between hardware and software. The rules of function are the rules of architecture, and function governs architecture, which governs function. We require a new vocabulary, a new set of concepts to replace the functionalist view. Several additional examples may extend our grasp of the emerging unity of structure and function, emphasize difficulties intrinsic to the functionalist program, and stress the need for new formulations.

Different experiences alter synaptic structure and function. Greenough and colleagues (1984) have found that exposure to an enriched environment increases synapse number in the cerebral cortex of adult rats. Perhaps more striking, performance of specific somatosensory tasks increases synapses in appropriate areas of the somatosensory cortex. A number of architectural features change: synapses per neuron increase, synapse density per unit volume rises, and dendritic (process) length increases. We shall certainly want to explore the relationship of environmental experience, neural architecture, and function in mammalian brain to begin understanding underlying, interrelating mechanisms.

The essential unity of structure and function, of hardware and software, is not restricted to mammals; it is evident in invertebrate nervous systems as well. For example, in the sea snail, *Aplysia californica*, the behavioral-physiological states, long-term habituation and sensitization, are associated with specific ultramicroscopic synaptic change (Bailey 1989). With habituation, in which physiological efficacy or efficiency of synaptic conduction decreases, active synaptic zone number, active zone area, and number of transmitter storage vesicles per active zone all decrease. These ultramorphologic traits increase in sensitization, in which synaptic efficacy increases. The number of varicosities, sites that contain synapses, parallel the synaptic changes in both habituation and sensitization. Moreover, the changes parallel the duration of change in the appropriate memory behaviorally. In sum, microarchitecture, physiological function, behavior, and "mental state" are aspects of the same neural processes in phylogenetically diverse forms. Functionalism is as inadequate to the task of explaining invertebrate behavior as that of complex mammals.

These few examples, drawn from a vast and growing literature, suggest that explanations of behavior, neurophysiological function, and the regulation of architecture will prove to be one in the same. And the explanatory language will be that of transmitter signals, growth factors, synaptic communication, architecture from the molecule to the system, and the resultant behavior and mental state. The program, the software, simply does not exist outside the biology of the nervous system.

The Connectionist Program: A Response to Functionalism

Functionalism arose as one solution to the perceived division of labor problem between a psychology focusing on mentation and behavior and a neuroscience pursuing neurobiologic mechanism. Functionalism and the dominant computer metaphor arose in the 1950s and has held sway since the 1970s. Nevertheless, even within psychology proper, doubts began emerging in the 1980s. The latent awareness that architecture does matter became manifest. For example, new and different procedures and algorithms are required for digital and analogue computers. The attempt to substitute the brain metaphor for the computer metaphor led to an approach termed the connectionist program (Rumelhart and McClelland 1986).

The central assumption of this approach is that knowledge exists in the connections, the pattern of connectivity among neurons. Learning consists of modification of connections, and therefore the principles of the regulation of connection are critical. In practice, the connectionist approach has focused on the computational aspects of connectivity in an effort to model psychobiology. However, in fact, connectionism has been largely preoccupied with only certain types of constraint and only certain aspects of biology.

The so-called real-time constraints are severe (Newell 1980). Information-processing elements in computers function in the nanosecond range (billionth of a second), while neurons function in the millisecond (thousandth of a second) range. This consideration alone suggests that the brain comprises a radically different design from the classical von Neumann computer. Even massively parallel neuronal architectures encounter extreme difficulties processing information in less than 1 or 2 seconds. Devising appropriate algorithms to simulate brain function while honoring the real-time constraint has been a major hurdle.

Another constraint derives from the sheer number of processing elements in the brain: approximately 100 billion neurons and 10^{15} synapses. Any plausible model of the brain must accommodate this complexity. Yet existing computational simulations are generally composed of tens of units, presumably representing individual neurons. Certainly it will be critical to determine explicitly whether computational elements in models represent synapses, neurons, neuronal assemblies, or even multiple systems before homologies or analogies to brain can be seriously entertained.

The connectionist, as the name implies, stresses the primacy of altering neuronal connections as the mechanisms underlying learning and memory. The neurobiologist has documented the growth of new connections, loss of old connections, and modification of existing connections in the living nervous system. The connectionist models only the last alternative, thereby ignoring some of the most important processes actually transpiring in the nervous system. Acknowledging the importance of simplification and idealization in model construction, it will be important to determine whether real brain function can be adequately simulated by ignoring critical biologic processes.

The connectionist program views learning as the optimization of local function procedures that maximize a global function of the network. What is the substance of the local (presumably neuronal and synaptic) processes that alter global function? I develop the view that *au/lw* it is precisely the changes in transmitter metabolism, expression and communication, alteration of synaptic molecular architecture, and modified growth and trophic factor action that constitute the biology of learning, memory, and neurologic function. Consequently we examine underlying mechanisms in detail to characterize constraints and understand features of cognitive function conferred by the biology of the living nervous system.

plural a weak

Reductionist Programs *there are 2 — extreme*

In general terms, the reductionist stance represents the polar opposite of functionalism. However, any discussion of reductionism must recognize that the term has been used to denote very different intellectual positions. The general, or weak, reductionist position differs radically *① def* from extreme reductionism. General reductionism holds that mind function is ultimately explicable in terms of physical structure and function of the brain; however, it makes no assumption about the salient levels of physical mechanism. Thus, genes, molecules, cells, populations, systems, system aggregates, epigenetic signals, behavior, mentation, and environmental mechanism, among others, are all of potential interest to the general reductionist. No level of function is excluded on a priori grounds by the general reductionist.

In contrast, extreme reductionism adopts the view that specific biological domains are of particular importance. While this stance seems to be a minor, quantitative variant of general reductionism, it leads to rather implausible positions. In its late twentieth-century form, the extreme position reduces focus to genes, molecules, and, at the limit, cells. The most radical position suggests that brain function can be comprehended in terms of gene expression and action. Genes contain the blueprint for the construction and function of the nervous system; a complete description of gene action will suffice to explain brain and mind function.

HPPNT

The extreme position ignores the centrality of cell, population, and systems organization, of architecture, in brain function. In an organ system devoted to communication in which communication **is** representation, architecture is function. Genes are informative only in the *context* of brain structure and function. An example drawn from clinical neurology may be illustrative. The Lesch-Nyhan syndrome is characterized by mental retardation and self-mutilation in children. The defective gene has been identified in this genetic disorder (Caskey 1987). Moreover, the specific DNA sequence abnormalities have been defined, and specific defective gene products have been isolated. Even the function of the faulty gene product is known. The gene product is an enzyme involved in purine metabolism, HPRT (hypoxanthine phosphoribosyltransferase). In spite of this detailed genetic and molecular information, we do not have the slightest insight into the mechanisms leading to mental retardation and self-mutilation. To approach these issues, we must frame questions in neurophysiological, neuroanatomical, and behavioral terms. The genetic defect has meaning only in the context of brain function. While this statement seems to be trivially obvious, entire research programs ignore this point. This example indicates the futility of considering gene function outside the context of brain organization. Gene structure and function are informative, in the present instance, only within the setting of neurobiological questions. What is the neuroanatomy and systems physiology of self-mutilation? Indeed, what is the appropriate place of self-mutilation in the taxonomy of behaviors, and neural systems, involved in grooming, self-image, self-awareness, and stereotypy, for example? Are these categories even relevant? What is the relevant neurobiology of mental retardation? The meaning of the genetic defect cannot be approached in the absence of this basic neurobiological information. While knowledge of the genetic and molecular biochemical deficits is necessary to understand mechanisms in the Lesch-Nyhan syndrome, this knowledge alone is insufficient. This simple example illustrates the impoverished nature of the extreme reductionist approach.

Another example, drawn from a radically different organism, further illustrates the inadequacy of the extreme reductionist formulation. Isogenic individuals of the species *Daphnia magna*, aquatic fleas, exhibit well-documented differences in structure of the nervous system. That is, genetically identical organisms have different nervous systems. For example, the pattern of axon branching of ommatidial receptor neurons of the optic ganglia differ among genetically identical individuals (Macagno et al. 1973). Indeed, each individual organism is different, although all are genetically the same. Needless to say, then, in outbred species, from locust to primate (Goodman et al. 1979; Kaas et al. 1983), nervous system structure differs markedly among individuals. Now, the reductionist of any stripe views the nervous system as the basis of behavior and any form of mental function; the extreme reductionist views genes as the unit of function. Consequently, extreme reductionism is presented with the paradox of invoking genes as the complete story specifying behavior based on neural structure, yet identical genetic constitutions result in dissimilar nervous systems. Therefore genes cannot comprise the complete account, and extreme reductionism is incomplete.

At this early stage of our inquiry, it might be useful to explicitly define the fatal problem of extreme reductionism. The difficulty lies not in the logic of seeking the basis of function in neural structure. Rather, the problem lies in assuming a restrictive posture that limits relevant structure to genes. As we proceed, we shall see that critical structures exist at multiple levels of organization of the nervous system—from gene to molecule to organelle, cell, system, network, behavior, and environment—and focus may be fruitfully directed to any single level, as an exemplar, **in the context of the nervous system as a whole.**

The latter, simplifying strategy is adopted by weak reductionism. The effort involves identification of scientifically tractable structural elements that process information in the nervous system. The set of elements is not assumed to account for brain function in its entirety. Rather, the goal is to define some of the principles that govern brain and mind function. The elements under study are regarded as relevant to the goal only in the context of the intact nervous system. It is the explicit burden of the experimentalist or theorist to insist on physiological context. Any set of elements is relevant only insofar as it processes information and simultaneously participates in ongoing neural function; these dual roles require the neural context.

Structure and Function in Brain and Mind

What structural elements may be usefully examined? It may be helpful to outline appropriate general characteristics before proceeding to more detailed discussions. A number of provisional requirements can be defined. First, neural elements of interest must change with environmental conditions. That is, environmental stimuli must, in some sense, regulate the function of these particular units such that the units actually serve to represent conditions of the real world. The potential units, or elements of interest, thereby function as symbols representing external or internal reality. The symbols, then, are actual physical structures that constitute neural language representing the real world. Symbolic function is a critical cornerstone, identifying neural structures of interest.

Second, the symbols must govern the function of the nervous system such that representation itself constitutes a change in neural state. Consequently symbols do not serve as indifferent repositories of information but govern ongoing function of the nervous system. Symbols in the nervous system simultaneously dictate the rules of operation of the system. In other words, the symbols are central to the architecture of the system; architecture confers the properties that determine behavior of the system. The syntax of symbol operation is the syntax of neural function. Syntactic structure allows for the combination of symbols to form more complex structures, which, in turn, lie at the heart of combinatorial capacity in mental function. Symbols of interest therefore possess structure, semantics, and syntactical relations, which are causally interrelated. We shall certainly want to identify functional loci in the nervous system where symbolic function fulfills these requirements.

Practically, it would be of great help to initially identify a relatively simple symbol domain to discern principles that may be applicable to far more complex spheres in the nervous system. Rather than beginning inquiry at the complicated level of networks of millions of neurons and billions of synapses, I attempt to adopt a simplifying approach. My goal is not to explain the complexity of brain function in its entirety in a single leap. Rather, I hope to decipher some of the rules of symbol structure and function at a simple level in preparation for more formidable tasks in the future.

Overview

My charge is to discuss the molecular and cellular biology of information processing in the nervous system. What molecular mechanisms allow neurons and their networks to learn from experience? Can we identify molecular loci where information processing transpires? In brief, do any molecular mechanisms receive, transduce, encode, store, retrieve, and express information about the real world? In approaching the central brain function of information processing, where might we fruitfully direct our focus?

One clue may derive from another central neural function, communication. With 100 billion neurons and approximately 10^{15} connections specialized for communication, the nervous system is clearly in the business of communication. We might guess that the two pivotal neural functions, communication and information processing, are integrally related. In fact, that is precisely the claim that I examine.

I discuss the proposition that the agents of communication, such as neurotransmitters, growth factors, and trophic factors, also process environmental information. We also examine the prime apparatus of communication, the synapse, to assess its role in information processing.

This inquiry encounters a multitude of fascinating processes. None is more remarkable than environmental regulation of neural function at perhaps the most fundamental level: gene action. That is, the environment, through impulse activity, accesses the genome, the blueprint for neural structure and function; the real world can model neural architecture at many levels of function simultaneously. Interaction with the environment elicits ongoing reorganization of the nervous system, and this dynamic process constitutes a central mechanism in information processing. Moreover, it is precisely communication through transmitter, growth factor, and trophic factor action that mediates continual neural remodeling. We examine the principles of biology underlying these processes to gain insights into rules governing resultant behaviors and mental states.

Finally, we examine the proposition that the very signals that communicate, that are responsible for millisecond-to-millisecond function, also process long-term information. We study the related contention that this class of molecular signals comprises one neural language encoding environmental information. The semantic and syntactic functions of these molecules are scrutinized in detail.

Communicative Symbols in the Nervous System

To begin approaching the biology of mental function, we focus on specific types of symbols in the nervous system. It may be useful to examine the simplest communicative symbols in the hope that general principles may be discerned. In turn, generalities emerging from consideration of simple symbols may be applicable to multiple cognitive functions in the nervous system. Can we define a relatively simple symbol set to serve as a prototype for other, more complicated sets in the nervous system?

In fact, certain molecules appear to function as communicative symbols. These molecules receive, transduce, store, and transmit information about the internal and external environments. These molecules form one potential biochemical basis for cognitive function. Even at the rudimentary, molecular level, critical cognitive functions are detectable. Which molecules are of particular interest?

I have already defined their character. The molecules of interest function symbolically and serve to communicate in the nervous system. We will focus on specific agents of communication: the neuro-transmitters, which convey impulses among neurons, and neurotrophic molecules, which help generate and maintain pathway connections. These agents of communication also receive, transduce, store, and transmit information in the nervous system. While we focus on transmitters almost exclusively, these elements simply serve as prototypes for simple, neural, information-bearing structures. Similar approaches may be applied to receptors, ion channels, and patterned impulse activity itself. Transmitters are employed as exemplars only, fully anticipating that other units may be analyzed in a parallel fashion.

It may be useful to emphasize this claim. I am suggesting that the molecules that carry out second-to-second function in the nervous system also serve cognitive, symbolic functions. The chemical signals crucial for ongoing communication in the brain also change function-ally with experience, leading to long-term changes associated with learning and memory. In other words, the nervous system uses certain molecules simultaneously as physiological signals and symbols, rep-resenting environmental information. This parsimonious principle of multiple function ensures that the environment simultaneously elicits appropriate physiologic responses and symbolic representation in the nervous system.

The principle of multiple function recurs at many levels of complex-ity in the nervous system. Different symbol sets serve multiple func-tions. If we can identify specific molecules that actually perform cognitive functions in the brain, we should want to know the rules that govern the action of these molecules. They may constrain and govern certain aspects of cognitive function. They may also affect function at other levels of neural organization, including synapses, neurons, and arrays of synapses and neurons. One goal of this book is to illustrate principles governing the actions and functions of the molecular, communicative symbols in the context of the nervous sys-tem. They help to explain a number of features of cognitive function. These principles help to explain how the brain can store information **about** something else. Moreover, knowledge of these principles indi-cates that symbols in the brain are both hardware and software and that these terms are actually misleading in understanding brain and behavior.

How do neural assemblies use molecules to implement cognitive strategies? How do these symbols participate in the conversion of the nearly endless array of real world information into neural language? We can use transmitters as prototypes to begin approaching the pro-cesses involved. (These are prototypes for other molecular symbols and for symbols in different domains as well, such as synaptic arrays.)

Two related strategies are employed by the nervous system in the manipulation of the transmitter molecular symbols. First, individual neurons use multiple transmitter signal types at any given time (for review, see Hokfelt et al. 1984). Second, each transmitter type may respond independently of others to environmental stimuli. Consequently a wide variety of transmitter ratios is available to the individual neuron to represent reality. This, then, is one set of mechanisms that allows the nervous system to convert a nearly endless array of real world information into neural language. How is this strategy useful?

The neuron appears to use a **combinatorial strategy,** a simple and elegant process used repeatedly in nature in a variety of guises. A series of distinct elements, of relatively restricted number, are used in a wide variety of combinations and permutations. For example, if a given neuron uses four different transmitters, and each can exist in only three different concentrations (based on environmental influences) independently, the neuron can exist in 3^4 discrete transmitter states. That is, the neuron is capable of existing in eighty-one different states in this particular example. However, this example appears to vastly underestimate combinatorial potential of the neuron in reality. Transmitters in the living neuron appear to be capable of existing in an extended number of states; the ultimate combinatorial potential of a neuron using only four transmitters may actually number in the hundreds. Estimates in the thousands may not be farfetched for many neurons. Indeed, if transmitters can exist in virtually continuous spectra of concentrations, combinatorial potentials may be virtually incalculable.

These considerations may be placed in the context of the nervous system. Complex mammalian systems consist of approximately 10^{11} or 100 billion neurons, each of which may exist in tens or hundreds of different transmitter states. Considering the unidimensional world of transmitters alone, the potential for information reception and storage is staggering. And we have not yet begun to examine other, independent mechanisms available for processing.

As we shall see, the transmitter symbols and combinatorial neurons are organized into complex pathways forming circuits of a particular character. The circuits are **electrochemically coded** (Bartfai et al. 1986). That is, electrical impulse activity of different frequencies and patterns releases specific transmitter combinations from particular neurons. This organization allows the performance of tasks that are critical for mental function, such as extraction of features from complex stimuli, completion of patterns from a fragment, and associational processing. Stated in the idiom already employed, the quality of aboutness or intentionality may well be approachable in terms of neuronal manipulation of transmitter symbols, combinatorial processing, and electro-chemical coding of neural circuits. We shall examine these processes in detail in subsequent chapters.

Temporal Dimension and Communicative Symbols

It is apparent that regulatory changes elicited by the environment occur over time. In a system concerned with the storage of information and with memory, this obvious fact could scarcely be of greater importance. I will continue to use the molecular transmitter symbols to illustrate this point preliminarily. Transmitter changes often last days to weeks in response to environmental stimuli lasting seconds to minutes (Zigmond 1989; Black 1975). These long-lasting transmitter changes form some of the basic units of memory mechanisms. Consequently even simple systems of neurons exhibit a rudimentary form of memory: **the temporal amplification of environmental information**. Based on this line of reasoning, we can see that memory at the molecular level is present in neurons throughout the nervous system; it is not restricted to a single brain center. The nervous system is not a simple computer containing a separate central processing unit and a memory. And transmitter symbols are both software and hardware, both structure and function. To understand molecular memory, we shall have to understand the rules that govern the change in transmitter status with time. Part of the book is devoted to this straightforward description.

Although I have identified some of the basic structures involved in memory, these processes do not account for long-term memory lasting years to decades. Other, virtually permanent changes must be involved. One clue to the potential nature of such long-term changes may come from understanding the mechanisms underlying the short- and intermediate-term changes. Current experiments indicate that transmitter changes are due to increased synthesis by the neuronal genome of messenger RNA encoding transmitters (Black et al. 1985; Biguet et al. 1986). We may speculate that stable alterations in gene action, elicited by environmental cues, contribute to long-term memory.

A second clue to mechanisms generating long-term memory comes from the discovery that experience, and use of a neural pathway, alters synaptic structure and function. That is, use in a particular manner alters both the signals that are sent and the molecular apparatus, the synapse, through which signals are sent. Moreover, preliminary evidence indicates that alteration in synaptic structure is longlasting, exhibiting the characteristics of long-term memory (Greenough 1984).

In turn, change in synaptic efficacy, or strength, alters transmission across a pathway in a quasi-permanent fashion, consistent with long-term memory.

The focus on the structural synapse, moreover, introduces another class of regulatory interactions—that governed by trophic molecules (Levi-Montalcini and Angeletti 1968). This class of endogenous factors appears to play a role in the growth of axons, the formation of synapses, and the maintenance of systems and synapses throughout life. Recent evidence suggests that trophic molecules may specifically regulate the molecular architecture of synapses, thereby influencing function. We shall certainly want to inquire about the role of synaptic structure, and that of trophic molecules, in the genesis of long-term memory.

Molecular Structures and Neural Systems Organization

Can we relate functional units to other cognitive functions? Can we move from molecular symbols to symbols at other levels of organization of the nervous system? One central concept to have emerged from extensive testing of humans and subhuman primates is that mental function is organized into "modules" (figure 1.1; see Gazzaniga 1989 for review). Cognition does not simply arise from a single, integrated system. Rather, different mental functions seem to operate independently within the individual. For example, in people, some agent in the (dominant) left cerebral hemisphere constantly makes up stories, theories, and hypotheses to explain external and internal reality. Even when deprived of sensory information, the "interpreter" in people continues to weave tales, now often inaccurate or blatantly incorrect, to account for a fragmented, discontinuous, perceived environment (Gazzaniga and LeDoux 1978). These and related observations have led cognitive psychologists to the concept that mind is composed of multiple, distinct mental modules. We may now ask whether these conceptual modules actually have a physical reality. The extraordinary, perhaps counterintuitive answer is "yes." At least some mental modules may be defined anatomically as neural subsystems in the brain. Further, these systems-modules exhibit distinctive molecular attributes. A single module may use the same transmitters and be dependent on common trophic agents. During development, the appropriate trophic molecules ensure formation of the subsystem, with its connections. During maturity, the trophic agents regulate function of the module and are necessary for maintenance of normal physiology. In other words, the scientific concept, psychologic modularity, appears to have a molecular, cellular, and systems reality. Subse-

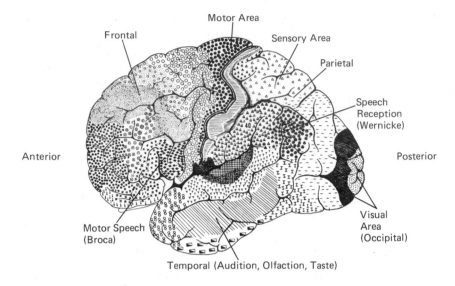

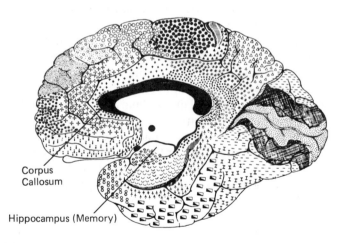

Figure 1.1
Schematic functional cytoarchitectural map of the human cerebral cortex. (From *Bing's Local Diagnosis in Neurological Diseases*, 1969; originally from Brodmann 1908)

quently we examine whether psychologic organization and functions can be driven "down" to the physical level. Indeed, psychology is not separable from the physical. Psychologic modular organization arises from physical modular organization. To understand mechanisms governing psychologic modularity, we must understand the physical modularity upon which psychology is based.

These observations illustrate several points. Functional structures are to be found in the psychologic as well as physical realms. In fact, clear distinctions between these realms will begin to blur as we proceed. It should be equally clear that symbolic function occurs from the molecular to psychologic domains, and these functions may be closely related. Finally, we can begin to see how derangement of modular function, at several different loci, may result in mental disease.

Mental Function and Cell Biology

This introductory sketch has been used to indicate that mentality may be fruitfully analyzed in terms of structural functional units. Even the simplest units, molecular symbols, receive, transduce, encode, store, and transmit information. Further, trophic molecules also help to create and maintain the neural systems, synaptic connections, and modules that actually give mental function its form. Remarkably, then, molecular symbols simultaneously mediate moment-to-moment communication, long-term information storage, and the formation of the very architecture of the nervous system. Transmitters function as signals and symbols subserving communication, embedded in the systems created and maintained by the trophic symbols. In fact, the distinction between transmitter and trophic agent is rapidly blurring. Molecular symbol, system, and behavior are inseparable. There is no hardware-software divide.

Cognitive function cannot be separated from the nervous system in which it is instantiated. Finally, the quality of aboutness is derived from the function of interacting communicative symbols in the molecular, synaptic, neuronal, network, and multisystems domains.

The foregoing arguments present a very general, even licentious overview of a monstrously complex topic. These telegraphic overviews present but skeletal arguments without the substantiating evidence and logical development that represent the spirit of this inquiry. The experimental observations, case histories, analyses, and syntheses that breathe life into these dry conjectures comprise the chapters of this book.

A Note about Subsequent Chapters and Organization

Before discussing molecular symbols in detail, it may be helpful to outline the traditional biochemical view of the synapse, the communicative junction between neurons. This conventional framework, presented in chapter 2, provides a basis for appreciation of emerging, novel formulations. Moreover, the background material also introduces the uninitiated to the basic language of neurochemistry, neuropharmacology, and the study of neurotransmitters. The chapter may also constitute a useful brief review for experienced neuroscientists as well. The classical knowledge provides the perspective, the context for the new information regarding co-transmitters, neuropeptides, modulation, gene expression, second messengers, and neural plasticity that have revolutionized our ability to relate molecules, behavior, and mental state. The new information is presented in subsequent chapters, after delineation of the orthodox formulation in the next chapter.

Chapter 2

A General Introduction to a Specific Synapse:

Definitions and Explanations

Historical Perspective—Catecholaminergic Synapse —Transmitter Synthesis, Storage, and Release—Receptor Adaptation—Presynaptic Autoreceptors and Unconventional Communication—Termination of Transmitter Action —Transmitter Phenotypic Expression—Coexpression of Transmitters—Long-Term Synaptic Change—Synaptic Plasticity— Postsynaptic Density—Long-Term Potentiation-NMDA Receptors

The traditional biochemical view of the synapse focuses on specific molecules, such as transmitters, receptors, and ion channels to identify loci of millisecond-to-millisecond communication. In addition, however, since the pioneering work of Hebb in 1949, the synapse, as the communicative junction between neurons, has assumed primacy in most formulations of the biology of learning and memory. Before considering some of the emerging concepts of synaptic function, it may be helpful to outline the classical knowledge to provide perspective and context.

Rather than discuss a variety of different synapses, we focus on a single, prototypical synapse that has played a pivotal role in the emergence of understanding. Synapses that use catecholamine (CA) neurotransmitters as signals, the subject of study for nearly a century, have yielded extensive insight into the nature of communication in the nervous system (for review, see Molinoff and Axelrod 1971). The very concept of chemical synaptic transmission (communication) was initially proposed for CA systems in 1905, with the postulate that an adrenaline (epinephrine)-like substance was released by terminals in the sympathetic nervous system, mediating physiological effects (Elliot 1905). The subsequent work of von Euler and colleagues established that the CA norepinephrine (NE) was the transmitter in question (for review, see Euler 1959). In another landmark advance, the introduction of a fluorescent method for the in situ histochemical visualization of the CAs, dopamine (DA), NE, and epinephrine (E), allowed confirmation of the earlier biochemical studies and permitted the first definition of transmitter-specific pathways in the central nervous system (CNS) (Falck et al. 1962). The recent availability of immunocytochemical methods for the visualization of CA biosynthetic enzymes has extended these observations and provided insights into the regulation of individual transmitter molecular traits (for review, see Black 1982).

In yet another sphere, the discovery of nerve growth factor (NGF), which enhances survival, development, and function of sympathetic CA neurons (as well as central neurons), has led to the first complete characterization of a neuronal trophic factor (see subsequent chapters for a review). Finally, the study of CA systems has been of prime importance in establishing that neurons may utilize more than one transmitter at any one time and that transmitters may change over time (for review, see Hokfelt et al. 1986). In summary, an understanding of CA regulatory processes has been central to an appreciation of synaptic function.

Before proceeding to more detailed discussion, it may be useful to address several general prefatory questions: What are CAs, where do they occur, and what do they do? DA, NE, and E are 3,4-dihydroxy derivatives of phenylethylamine (figure 2.1) and are localized to peripheral sympathetic neurons, the adrenal medulla and other peripheral aggregates of chromaffin tissue, and a number of discrete brainstem nuclei that project throughout the neuraxis. It is evident,

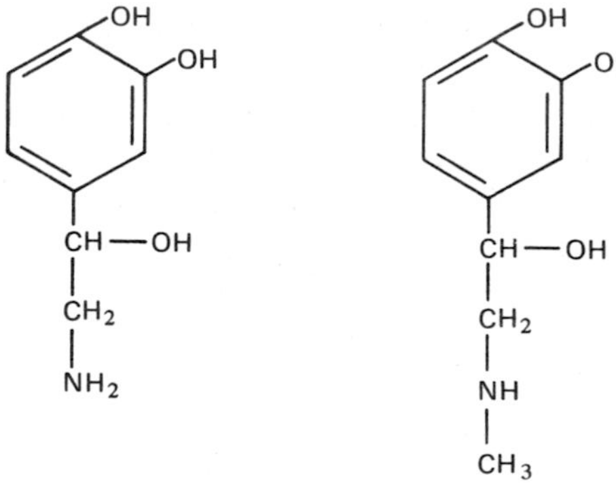

Norepinephrine   Epinephrine

Figure 2.1
Biochemical structure of two important catecholamines. Note the adjacent hydroxyl (-OH), catechol group on the benzene ring, the betahydroxyl group, and the distinguishing amine group.

therefore, that the CAs may alter function of a wide variety of cell and tissue types, including vascular smooth muscle, heart, liver, adipocytes, and a multiplicity of brain neurons. CA effects are mediated by interaction with specific postsynaptic receptors, frequently eliciting changes in postsynaptic adenylate cyclase, 3', 5'-cAMP, and postsynaptic proteins (for review, see Greengard 1976). This sequence of events at the molecular level may result in such varied physiologic responses as tachycardia, peripheral vasoconstriction, mydriasis, and inhibition of peristalsis. Central CA systems are critical for normal motor control and have been implicated in a variety of neuropsychiatric diseases, including Parkinson's disease and affective disorders (Cotzias et al. 1969; Schildkraut and Kety 1967). Indeed, the study of CA synapses and transmitters has yielded some of the most useful molecular-physiologic-behavioral correlations available in neuroscience.

To define mechanisms underlying the function of CA synapses, this very brief summary follows the transmitter molecule itself as it is sequentially processed inside and outside the nerve terminal (figure 2.2). Initially, CA biosynthesis is described, with particular emphasis on regulatory mechanisms. Subsequent sections deal with processes governing CA storage, release, interaction with receptors, and termination of action. Regulation of CA phenotypic expression and other putative transmitters in catecholaminergic neurons is described. A number of relatively recent reviews are recommended (Iversen 1967; Molinoff and Axelrod 1971; Moore and Bloom 1978, 1979).

Biosynthesis

CAs are synthesized from dietary tyrosine by a series of enzymes, which, in turn, are themselves synthesized within perikarya and transported distally to axon terminals (figure 2.3). Physiologically active CA is synthesized and stored within the nerve terminal. NE is synthesized within sympathetic neurons in the periphery, whereas E is the predominant amine in the adrenal medulla. DA, NE, and E all appear to function as transmitters in different central neuronal systems. DA is utilized by the nigro-striatal and mesencephalic-cortical systems (Moore and Bloom 1978). NE is highly localized to the pontine nucleus locus coeruleus, which projects to the cerebral and cerebellar cortices, as well as the spinal cord (Moore and Bloom 1979). Finally, E has been identified in a number of nuclei in the medulla oblongata, which may subserve visceral regulatory functions (Moore and Bloom 1979). In spite of this geographic and functional heterogeneity, the CAs are predominantly synthesized by a single biochemical pathway.

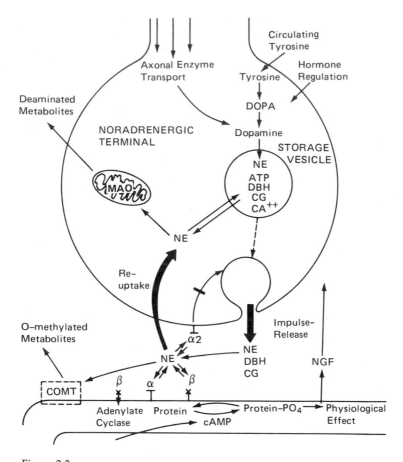

Figure 2.2
The catecholaminergic synapse. A terminal or "varicosity" of a norepinephrine-containing neuron is pictured above, and the postsynaptic target cell is pictured below. The general scheme for the biosynthesis and regulation of the norepinephrine transmitter is depicted.
NE = norepinephrine; ATP = adenosinetriphosphate; DBH = dopamine-β-hydroxylase; CG = chromogranin; Ca^{++} = calcium ion; NGF = nerve growth factor; pre- and postsynaptic receptors are denoted by Greek letters.

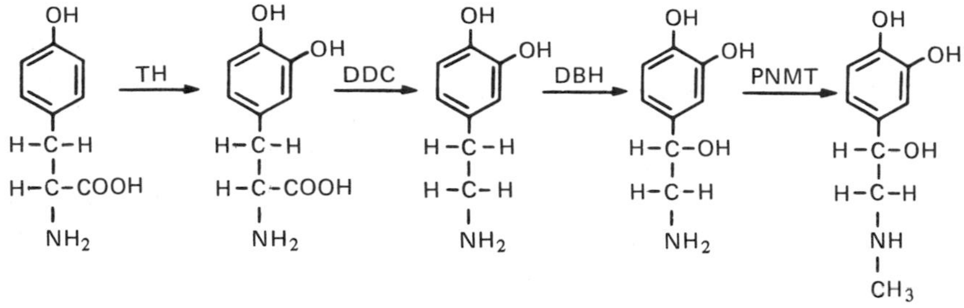

Tyrosine L-Dopa Dopamine Norepinephrine Epinephrine

Figure 2.3
Catecholamine biosynthesis.
TH = tyrosine hydroxylase; DDC = DOPA decarboxylase, also known as L-aromatic amino acid decarboxylase; DBH = dopamine-β-hydroxylase; PNMT = phenylethanolamine-N-methyltransferase.

Tyrosine hydroxylase, the rate-limiting enzyme in CA biosynthesis (Levitt et al. 1965), converts tyrosine to L-DOPA. This cytoplasmic, pteridine-requiring enzyme is dependent on Fe^{++} and O_2 for maximal activity and is subject to both short- and long-term regulation. It is subject to (rapid) feedback inhibition by DA and NE, products of the CA biosynthetic pathway itself (for review see Molinoff and Axelrod 1971, figure 2.3). Long-term regulation is achieved through biochemical induction, increasing the number of enzyme molecules present in the cell. In sympathetic neurons and perhaps in central NE neurons as well (for review, see Molinoff and Axelrod 1971), increased neuronal firing leads to enzyme induction. In the peripheral sympathetics, the increase in neuronal activity appears to be mediated by presynaptic cholinergic neurons, leading to the presumption that this represents an instance of "transsynaptic enzyme induction."

In addition to regulating CA biosynthesis under normal physiologic conditions, tyrosine hydroxylase may be manipulated experimentally to radically alter the state of CA neurons. For example, administration of α-methyl-p-tyrosine, a competitive inhibitor of the enzyme, causes selective depletion of peripheral and central CAs. The experimental and clinical utility of such an approach need not be stressed.

L-DOPA, formed by the hydroxylation of tyrosine, is converted to DA by L-aromatic amino acid decarboxylase (DOPA decarboxylase). This ubiquitous enzyme is endowed with minimal substrate specificity, as the name implies. Moreover, it is not induced by transsynaptic stimulation, which induces tyrosine hydroxylase (Black et al. 1971). Nevertheless, this enzyme has assumed increased clinical importance with the development of L-DOPA therapy for Parkinson's disease. Inhibitors of the enzyme, which do not cross the blood-brain barrier, are routinely administered with L-DOPA to increase delivery of the amine to nigro-striatal neurons by inhibiting peripheral decarboxylation.

DA, formed by decarboxylation, is concentrated by CA storage vesicles and converted to NE by intravesicular dopamine-β-hydroxylase. This enzyme, like tyrosine hydroxylase, is subject to transsynaptic induction in sympathetics and the adrenal. This Cu^{++}-containing enzyme is inhibited by disulfiram, which may chelate Cu^{++} in vivo and thereby deplete NE and E (for review, see Molinoff and Axelrod 1971).

The final step in CA biosynthesis, which occurs in the adrenal medulla and in some neuronal groups of the medulla oblongata, is catalyzed by phenylethanolamine-N-methyltransferase (PNMT). This enzyme methylates a variety of phenylethanolamines in addition to NE. Like tyrosine hydroxylase, PNMT is subject to inhibition by its product (in this case E). Moreover, PNMT in the adrenal is also induced by transsynaptic stimulation. In addition, adrenal PNMT is critically dependent on glucocorticoids and the pituitary-adrenal axis. Hypophysectomy results in a profound decrease in adrenal PNMT activity, which may be prevented or reversed by the administration of ACTH or glucocorticoids (for review, see Molinoff and Axelrod, 1971). Recent work suggests that the glucocorticoid-dependent developmental increase in PNMT molecules is mediated by an increase in messenger RNA coding for synthesis of the enzyme (Sabban et al. 1982). (The role of glucocorticoids in the regulation of brain PNMT has yet to be elucidated fully.) In summary, PNMT represents one locus at which the endocrine system directly influences CA biosynthesis. While glucocorticoids also increase sympathetic tyrosine hydroxylase activity, this effect requires intact presynaptic innervation and may therefore involve indirect transsynaptic mechanisms.

To summarize, tyrosine hydroxylase, dopamine-β-hydroxylase, and PNMT catalyze critical steps in CA biosynthesis, and all three enzymes are subject to complex regulatory mechanisms.

More generally, regulation of transmitter synthesis shares important commonalities in neurons that differ functionally, anatomically, and embryologically. This point is worthy of emphasis. Increased impulse activity stimulates transmitter synthesis in dopaminergic nigral neurons that regulate coordination of motor function, noradrenergic locus coeruleus neurons that may play a critical role in attention and arousal, and adrenergic adrenomedullary cells central to the stress response. Simply stated, the common biochemical and genomic organization of these diverse populations determines how environmental, epigenetic information, through altered impulse activity, is translated into neural information. In this prototypical example, cellular biochemical organization, not behavioral modality, is a key determinant of how external stimuli are converted to neural language. In this domain, modes of information storage are biochemically specific, not modality specific, indicating that synaptic systems subserving entirely different behavioral and cognitive functions may share common modes of information processing.

Storage

Subsequent to synthesis, CAs are stored within membrane-bound vesicles, which simultaneously protect the amines from enzymatic destruction and inactivate them. The CA storage vesicles, or granules, are predominantly of two types: peripheral sympathetic vesicles are 400–600Å in diameter, whereas adrenomedullary chromaffin granules are 100Å. Both have dense cores on electron microscopy. The vesicles concentrate CAs against a gradient, and this process requires Mg^{++} and ATP and is temperature dependent. The vesicles contain ATP, dopamine-β-hydroxylase, and a group of proteins designated chromogranins. Although the precise molecular mechanisms mediating vesicular uptake and storage have yet to be elucidated fully, a number of experimentally useful approaches are available.

Many phenylethylamine derivatives, such as tyramine and amphetamine, release physiologically active NE from vesicles, thereby eliciting a variety of CA effects. On the other hand, reserpine interferes with vesicular CA storage, but the amines are immediately inactivated by enzymatic deamination, resulting in depletion centrally and peripherally. The vesicles also concentrate exogenous compounds, such as α-methylnorepinephrine, which exhibit only a fraction of the potency of native NE. The normal transmitter may thereby be displaced by the analogue, which, in turn, is released upon neuronal discharge. This "false transmitter" markedly attenuates the effects of nerve stimulation (for a classical review of the area of storage, see Iversen 1967).

Release

Upon nerve stimulation, CAs are released along with ATP, dopamine-β-hydroxylase, and chromogranins, the other vesicular contents, suggesting that exocytosis underlies release. Moreover, as in the case of other transmitters and hormones, Ca^{++} is required, further suggesting that a number of common mechanisms govern release of diverse biologic signals.

For NE-containing nerves, stimulus-release relationships describe a rectangular hyperbole in which small changes in stimulation frequency, below approximately 5 per second, result in large changes in CA released (Mellander 1960). In fact, the normal rate of discharge is generally thought to be in the range of 1–2 per second. Considerable evidence suggests that stimulation preferentially releases newly synthesized NE. It is not yet clear, however, whether such a kinetically defined pool of NE corresponds to a particular spatial distribution of NE within the nerve terminal.

A variety of drugs, characterized structurally by a highly basic center linked by a one- or two-carbon chain to a ring, are capable of blocking CA release. Such agents as bretylium and guanethidine are particularly potent and have been used experimentally. Other compounds, the false transmitters, reduce the amount of transmitter released by displacement within the storage vesicle (see Iversen 1967 for review).

Recently a novel series of mechanisms regulating transmitter release has been posited as the basis of short- and long-term memory of sensitization of a specific defensive withdrawal reflex in the sea snail (Kandel and Schwartz 1982). In brief, experiments suggest that stimulation by serotonin elicits presynaptic facilitation of transmitter release, resulting in sensitization (figure 2.4). In this scenario, stimulation by serotonin increases intraneuronal cAMP, the classic second messenger, which, through a series of reactions (see figure 2.4), inactivates a novel K+ channel, thereby slowing depolarization of the action potential, allowing more Ca^{++} to flow into the nerve terminal. Ca^{++} influx increases transmitter release, resulting in sensitization. The critical biochemical reactions may involve phosphorylation of the appropriate ion channels by protein kinases, using cAMP. The central point for this discussion is that this represents a specific set of molecular mechanisms through which altered transmitter release may directly govern information flow in a simple nervous system.

It is apparent that multiple presynaptic mechanisms, from the regulation of synthesis to the regulation of release, may store information in the neuron at the synapse.

Catecholamine Receptors

CAs exert physiologic effects by interacting with specific receptors on the postsynaptic, target cell membrane, frequently altering concentrations of the second messenger, cAMP, thereby eliciting selective pro-

Presynaptic terminal

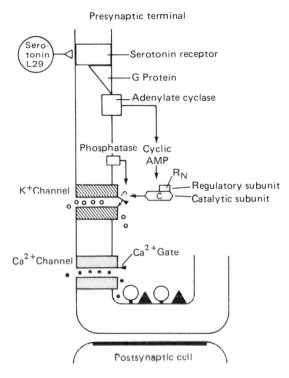

Figure 2.4
A proposed molecular model of presynaptic facilitation that may underlie the phenomenon of sensitization. (After Kandel and Schwarz 1982)

tein phosphorylation. CA receptors have been subdivided into two types, based on agonist potency: for α-receptors NE > E >> isoproterenol (ISO), whereas for β-receptors, ISO > E > NE (Ahlquist 1948). In general terms, both receptor types may be present within a single tissue, and excitatory or inhibitory effects do not simply correlate with receptor type. α-receptor stimulation results in such peripheral effects as vasoconstriction, uterine contraction, and mydriasis, while β-receptors mediate vasodilation, inhibition of uterine contraction, cardiac stimulation, and bronchodilation. With the availability of increasingly specific ligands, it has become apparent that receptors may be further subdivided into subtypes. Different subtypes are located in different structures and mediate different physiologic effects (for review see Minneman et al. 1981). Moreover, some receptors are located on the presynaptic membrane. For example, α-receptors are presynaptic and inhibit NE release when stimulated, constituting a negative feedback mechanism. These have been termed autoreceptors (Langer 1974). Finally, it is now apparent that DA receptors in the brain represent a different type, and recent studies suggest that they are composed of different subtypes as well (Huff and Molinoff 1982).

A number of molecular mechanisms modulate receptor number and the affinity of receptor binding. For example, in the presence of guanosine triphosphate (GTP), only low-affinity CA binding is apparent in the case of β-receptors, and this effect may be mediated by a GTP-binding protein coupled to the receptor. In another example, prolonged exposure to an agonist results in desensitization (tolerance) because of initial reduced affinity of the receptor for agonist and a subsequent decrease in receptor number, termed down-regulation. Conversely, denervation, CA depletion, or treatment with CA antagonists may lead to suprasensitivity because of an increase in receptor number. Even from this very brief survey, it is apparent that a variety of regulatory mechanisms at the receptor level may profoundly alter responses of the postsynaptic cell to presynaptic stimulation.

What are some of the cellular responses mediated by stimulation of noradrenergic receptors? One model system employed extensively is the noradrenergic locus coeruleus in the rostral pons and one set of its target neurons, the cerebellar Purkinje cells (for review see Moore and Bloom 1979). Extensive studies suggest that stimulation of Purkinje β-receptors by coeruleal NE depresses spontaneous discharge of Purkinje cells. Iontophoretic application of NE to Purkinje cells, or coeruleal stimulation elicits hyperpolarization with either no alteration or an increase in membrane resistance. β-receptor antagonists block the response to NE. Moreover, cAMP application reproduces the effects of NE, suggesting that release of NE by coeruleal terminals stimulates Purkinje β-receptors, with a resultant increase in cAMP and membrane hyperpolarization. It is not yet clear whether phosphorylation of critical postsynaptic proteins mediates this effect.

Although a great deal of detailed information concerning receptor types, structure, and kinetics is available, we now focus on a remarkable regulatory mechanism of import: receptor adaptation. Receptor adaptation allows the postsynaptic cell to detect minute changes in the **relative** concentrations of transmitter over time while reducing sensitivity to absolute levels at any instant. Consequently the postsynaptic cell can detect and respond to tiny changes in presynaptic impulse frequency but adapts to a constant rate of firing through mechanisms with varying time constants. How is this accomplished at the molecular level?

Catecholamine receptor number (B_{max}) and affinity for transmitter (K_d) are inversely related to transmitter concentrations in the synaptic cleft (figure 2.2). Elevation of transmitter concentration acutely activates receptors through direct binding and then decreases subsequent binding to the same receptors. Conversely reduction of transmitter acutely decreases receptor activation but then results in elevated receptor binding. The receptor system is thus organized to detect **changes** in transmitter concentration (and therefore presynaptic activity) as opposed to absolute concentration. Prolonged exposure to transmitter (or agonist) results in desensitization (tolerance) due to a rapid, reduced **affinity** of the receptor for agonist binding occurring over seconds and a subsequent decrease in receptor **number** over hours to days, termed down-regulation. On the other hand, catecholamine depletion, frank denervation, or treatment with catecholamine antagonists leads to suprasensitivity because of an increase in receptor number.

Molecular mechanisms underlying receptor adaptation have been defined in detail only for several receptor subtypes; nevertheless, the basic principles appear to be universal for transmitter receptor systems. The biologic strategy is to detect change from current levels of stimulation, whether up or down. Change in stimulus frequency is detected, noted, and rapidly discounted, enabling the next change to be detected. In essence, receptor systems are designed to detect changes in the neuronal environment at the expense of monitoring the status quo precisely. This fundamental principle is as true of receptors in the cerebral cortex as of receptors in the peripheral sympathetic nervous system.

Further, alteration of receptor number, whether up-regulation or down-regulation, persists for days after transmitter concentrations have returned to normal, basal levels. Consequently the transmitter apparatus exhibits **temporal amplification,** reminiscent of the properties of the biosynthetic system. Once again, a neural molecular system exhibits the ability to transduce, encode, and store information.

Presynaptic Receptors: Unconventional Communication

Relatively recently it became apparent that receptors are not restricted to the postsynaptic membrane but are also present on the presynaptic membrane (figure 2.2; Langer 1974). Activation of these receptors alters the subsequent release of transmitter by the presynaptic neuron. For example, one subtype of catecholaminergic receptor, the α-2 receptor, is located on sympathetic noradrenergic nerve terminals. Norepinephrine released by the neuron itself binds to the α-2 receptors, which results in decreased subsequent release of transmitter. In this manner, the neuron monitors its own activity and regulates transmitter released through a negative feedback mechanism. The neuron communicates with itself through stimulation of these "autoreceptors." It is unclear whether autocommunication elicits other, unrecognized, long-lasting effects in the neuron or at the synapse. Unexpectedly, noncatecholaminergic receptors have also been localized to the presynaptic noradrenergic terminal membrane. For example, angiotensin II receptors on the membrane also modulate norepinephrine release. Angiotensin is a potent vasoconstrictor, derived from circulating angiotensinogen by the action of renin, an enzyme secreted by the kidney (juxtaglomerular apparatus). While the detailed mechanisms are interesting, the principle is startling: the kidney can communicate with sympathetic neurons through nonsynaptic mechanisms. In a sense, in this instance, the neuron is an endocrine target. Circulating hormone regulates transmitter release at the synapse. Synaptic communication, then, may be modulated by nonsynaptic mechanisms, and distant structures may talk to receptive neurons. Consequently aspects of **communication with the nervous system are freed from hard-wiring constraints.**

In summary, presynaptic receptors serve proximate and distant communication and provide precision in the regulation of synaptic communication. In a critical sense, the nervous system cannot be abstracted out of the rest of the body in which it exists. Psychosomatic function thus assumes a specific somatic-neural, as well as neural-somatic, mechanistic reality, definable in molecular terms. Somatic and neural experiences are converted into altered neural biology, a recurrent theme in our inquiry.

Termination of Catecholamine Action

Rapid termination of transmitter action is of critical importance to synaptic function, allowing maximal information flow during interneuronal communication. CAs are predominantly inactivated by uptake into the presynaptic nerve terminal itself (for review see Iversen 1967). This high-affinity, saturable, stereospecific, energy-requiring process is capable of concentrating NE against a gradient of 10,000 to 1. It follows that any condition that inhibits uptake will markedly accentuate and prolong the effects of CA stimulation. This is precisely the effect of such drugs as desipramine and cocaine, highly specific inhibitors of uptake. It may be further inferred that in the absence of CA terminals, as in denervation, actions of exogenous amines are markedly intensified due to absence of uptake. This indeed is the case, indicating that denervation suprasensitivity is attributable to presynaptic as well as postsynaptic abnormalities.

Although neuronal uptake is the primary inactivating mechanism for CAs, enzymes that metabolize the amines have been identified and characterized. Catechol-O-methyltransferase (COMT) and monoamine oxidase (MAO) convert the CAs to physiologically inactive products (for review see Molinoff and Axelrod 1971). MAO actually consists of several different mitochondrial enzymes, with differing substrate specificities, which oxidatively deaminate DA, NE, and E to form the corresponding aldehydes. The use of MAO inhibitors in vivo markedly increases intraneuronal concentrations of CAs and decreases excretion of deaminated metabolites such as 3-methoxy-4-hydroxyphenylglycol and 3-methoxy-4-hydroxymandelic acid. COMT, predominantly an extraneuronal enzyme, metabolizes NE and E to the corresponding 3-0-methylamines, normetanephrine and metanephrine, using s-adenosylmethionine as a methyl donor. This enzyme is primarily involved in the metabolism of CAs released into the circulation and is found in highest concentrations in the liver and kidney. COMT may also play a relatively important role in the metabolism of NE in tissues with a sparse catecholaminergic innervation.

Catecholamine Phenotypic Expression

It is apparent, even from this brief description, that the function of the catecholaminergic synapse depends on the normal expression of a variety of CA phenotypic characters. Biosynthetic and catabolic enzymes, proteins associated with storage vesicles, release and reuptake mechanisms, and autoreceptors, to cite obvious examples, must be appropriately expressed by the neuron to ensure normal synaptic function. How is the expression of these diverse traits coordinated? Although a comprehensive answer is not yet available, increasing evidence suggests that environmental information from a variety of sources regulates expression of neuronal transmitter characters. Most of the relevant studies have focused on peripheral noradrenergic neurons.

In the mature sympathetic neuron, CA phenotypic characters are expressed within precise basal limits. Orthograde transsynaptic factors, retrograde transsynaptic factors from targets, humoral factors, and nonneuronal support cell factors all appear to contribute to the maintenance of appropriate levels of CA phenotypic characters (for review, see Black 1982). For example, denervation (decentralization) of sympathetic ganglia results in decreased tyrosine hydroxylase activity due to a reduction in cholinergic, transsynaptic stimulation.

Conversely, postganglionic axotomy, which separates sympathetic neurons from targets, also reduces enzyme activity. This effect is prevented by treatment with the trophic protein, NGF, suggesting that targets elaborate NGF, which regulates phenotypic expression in the sympathetic neuron. The influence of hormones, such as glucocorticoids, has already been described. Finally, dissociation of sympathetic neurons from adult ganglia, and growth outside the normal milieu, results in the appearance of cholinergic characters within the neurons. These observations, in aggregate, illustrate the critical role played by the environment in the regulation of CA phenotypic expression in the mature neuron.

Analogous environmental regulatory mechanisms govern the ontogeny of CA phenotypic characters in the embryo, fetus, and neonate. For example, the embryonic microenvironment through which autonomic neuroblasts migrate, and the environment of the definitive site, appears to influence the choice of transmitter phenotype. Additionally, in dissociated cell culture, neurons express cholinergic and/or noradrenergic traits, depending on the culture environment. For example, depolarizing stimuli foster noradrenergic expression, whereas factor(s) produced by nonneuronal cells induce cholinergic properties. Moreover, dual-function, cholinergic-noradrenergic neurons have been observed (for review see Patterson 1978). Consequently it is apparent that neurons may express more than one transmitter phenotype at any time. In fact, recent work has suggested that the transmitter phenotype of CA neurons may vary throughout life, depending on environmental signals.

Coexpression of Catecholaminergic and Peptidergic Phenotypes

The foregoing observations raise the possibility that CA neurons express a number of different putative transmitters. In fact, recent studies suggest that peripheral sympathetic CA neurons also express the putative peptide transmitter, substance P (SP), under appropriate environmental conditions in vivo and in vitro (Black 1982; Kessler et al. 1981). SP is an undecapeptide heterogeneously distributed in the central and peripheral nervous systems. Considerable evidence suggests that the peptide may function as a transmitter in peripheral sensory neurons, mediating nociceptive transmission. It is now apparent that transsynaptic impulse activity in sympathetic ganglia regulates the expression of SP in CA neurons, in addition to regulation of CA phenotypic characters.

In adult and neonatal rats, presynaptic cholinergic fibers decrease SP in CA sympathetic perikarya through the mediation of transsynaptic acetylcholine and stimulation of postsynaptic, nicotinic receptors (Kessler et al. 1981). Moreover, this effect appears to be mediated by transmembrane Na^+ flux in the postsynaptic neurons, based on studies performed in culture. Explantation of ganglia to culture, with consequent denervation, results in more than a twenty-fold increase in SP within 24 hours. Veratridine, an alkaloid that depolarizes neurons by increasing trans-membrane Na^+ flux, blocks this rise; tetrodotoxin, a specific inhibitor of the Na^+ flux effects of veratridine, prevents the SP effects of the alkaloid. If neuronal depolarization decreases SP in sympathetic neurons, manipulations that increase impulse flow in the sympathetic system in vivo also might be expected to decrease the peptide. In fact, this is the case. It may be concluded that transsynaptic impulse flow, which induces postsynaptic CA enzymes, decreases SP. Consequently depolarization has opposite effects on SP and CAs in sympathetic neurons. In more general terms, it is apparent that the neurotransmitter(s) expressed by a neuron, quantitatively and perhaps qualitatively, reflect the physiologic state of the neuron. In turn, it is possible that the transmitter employed by a synapse may be dependent on the state of the neuron. In this sense, then, it may be misleading to refer to synapses as either catecholaminergic or peptidergic (or cholinergic), implying neurohumoral exclusivity. To the contrary, synapses may be endowed with the ability to use multiple transmitters or to change transmitters in a dynamic fashion, reflecting the physiologic state of the neuron. (The consequences of transmitter co-localization are discussed extensively in subsequent chapters. This summary represents a simplified, orienting overview.)

Long-Term Synaptic Change

Consideration of synaptic transmission has illustrated that the synapse is hardly a simple digital switch, enslaved to a few, simple physiological variables. Quite the opposite occurs. Synaptic communication is a remarkably flexible and changing process, subject to modification by intraneuronal, extraneuronal local microenvironmental and even distant regulatory mechanisms. Are we now in a position to understand how molecular transformations alter gross synaptic structure (observable morphology)?

It may be helpful to enunciate explicitly the disparate synaptic processes that we are attempting to interrelate in our efforts to understand some of the biological bases of cognitive function. How does presynaptic impulse activity and transmitter release, with consequent activation of postsynaptic receptors and depolarization through ion flux, result in quasi-permanent changes in synaptic structure that alters function over prolonged periods of time? This is a critical question since these processes appear to participate in many forms of learning and memory.

The postsynaptic density (PSD) is a structure that may play a central role in the transduction of synaptic molecular mechanisms into alterations of morphology and function of long duration. The PSD is a proteinaceous, disc-shaped structure that lies tightly apposed to the postsynaptic membrane of virtually all chemical synapses. The PSD is readily visualized with the electron microscope (figures 2.5, 2.6; for review, see Siekevitz 1985). The PSD is actually a complex supramolecular structure that contains many components that participate in synaptic transmission and may undergo long-term changes associated with learning and memory. Transmitter receptors, including, for example, beta-adrenergic, glutamate, and GABA (gamma-aminobutyric acid) receptors, are anchored to the PSD through the postsynaptic membrane (figure 2.6; Siekevitz 1985). Consequently the receptors are potentially in a position to alter PSD structure and function, a circumstance that will assume importance later in this discussion. Moreover, the PSD contains a group of filamentous proteins that are well known to undergo movement and that confer shape, suggesting that the PSD is capable of dynamic geometrical changes. Actin, one of the key motile proteins in muscle, is a major component of the PSD (for review see Siekevitz 1985). In addition, fodrin, an actin- and calmodulin-binding protein, is part of the PSD, also suggesting that the PSD is morphologically mutable. In this category, tubulin, a protein necessary for the normal morphology of nerves, is also localized to the PSD (figure 2.6). Last, the PSD appears to be bound to the **presynaptic membrane,** and perhaps the presynaptic transmitter vesicular matrix, by fibrous proteins that traverse the synaptic cleft. Potentially, then, the PSD may simultaneously regulate pre- as well as postsynaptic function.

Finally, a number of molecules capable of altering structure through chemical reactions are also integral parts of the PSD. For example, the protein kinase enzymes, which are activated by cyclic AMP (adenosine monophosphate) and Ca^{++}, are also components of the PSD. This is of particular significance since these enzymes, with different substrate specificities, phosphorylate different structural proteins associated with the PSD. And phosphorylation is one critical mechanism that alters three-dimensional structure of proteins, thereby altering geometry and function. In summary, the PSD is so constituted that depolarization, Ca^{++} flux, and phosphorylation may transmit information that alters the structure and function of this key synaptic structure.

We are now in a position to appreciate how, in principle, normal neural activity induces molecular changes that alter the structure and function of the synapse. Although specific molecular mechanisms may differ for different chemical synapses, a series of mechanisms has emerged for certain synapses that serve as prototypes for the manner in which long-term information may be stored, based on experience. The induction of LTP in the hippocampus, a structure long suspected of playing a role in storage of certain types of memories, may provide a useful model (Bliss and Lomo 1973; Lynch 1986; Nicoll et al. 1988). LTP is a long-lasting increase in synaptic strength of excitatory afferents to hippocampal neurons. It occurs consequent to high-frequency activation of the afferents with postsynaptic discharge. What mechanisms are involved?

The consensus hypothesis suggests that presynaptic release of the excitatory transmitter, glutamate, and activation of a particular type of postsynaptic receptor elicits LTP. The activation of N-methyl-D-aspartate (NMDA) receptors with the consequent entry of Ca^{++} into postsynaptic neurons appears to mediate LTP (Collingridge et al. 1983; for reviews, see Lynch 1986; Bear et al. 1987; Nicoll et al. 1988). Ca^{++} influx presumably activates Ca^{++}/calmodulin kinase enzymes, which may act on critical proteins in the PSD, thereby altering synaptic spine shape and resulting in long-lasting changes in synaptic efficacy (figure 2.7; Lynch and Baudry 1984; Siekevitz 1985). How might alteration in dendritic spine morphology strengthen localized synapses?

Alteration of spine shape may result in several significant changes simultaneously. First, it may result in the exposure of formerly hidden (occluded) NMDA receptors that strengthen postsynaptic responses to presynaptic glutamate (Lynch and Baudry 1984). Subsequent enhanced receptor activation serves to perpetuate and amplify these changes, resulting in the long-term changes associated with memory formation and the storage of information.

Second, altered shape appears to change the electrical properties of the spine, which change response properties. A variety of modeling experiments (for review, see Shepherd 1986) indicate that the spine neck (figure 2.7) exhibits extremely high electrical resistance that amplifies depolarization resulting from synaptic discharge at the spine head. Lengthening of the neck in response to afferent stimulation and altered PSD conformation may thereby permit increased Ca^{++} influx consequent to NMDA receptor activation. In summary, a series of molecular reactions, including NMDA receptor activation, Ca^{++} influx, and kinase activation, may result in altered dendritic spine morphology, which, in turn, strengthens synapses in a long-lasting manner. And this may constitute one critical step in the formation of

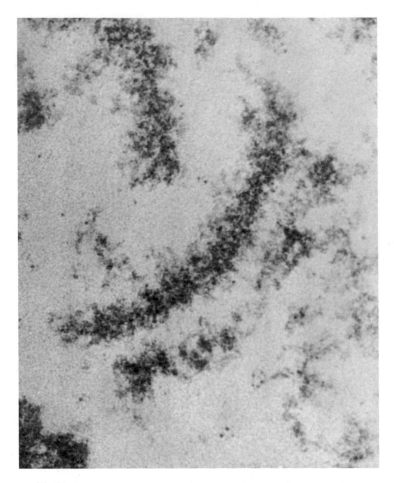

Figure 2.5
Electron micrograph of a postsynaptic density. Note the proteinaceous disc-shaped subcellular organelle, derived from the cerebral cortex, that is normally apposed to the inner surface of the postsynaptic membrane of chemical synapses. Magnification equals 26,000.

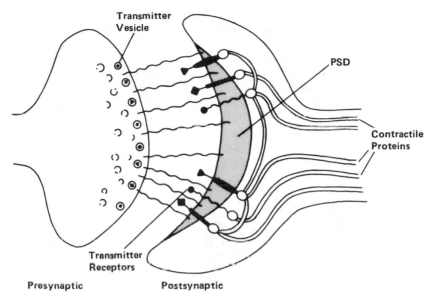

Figure 2.6
Schematic representation of a chemical synapse with the PSD in place. Alteration of the molecular structure of the PSD is thought to alter postsynaptic shape and thereby potentially alter long-term synaptic transmission.

memories by the hippocampus. Are these mechanisms relevant to other cortical areas that may participate in the storage of information? In fact, NMDA receptor stimulation and Ca^{++} influx appear to govern synaptic plasticity in the visual cortex that may be long lasting (Geiger and Singer 1984). It will now be important to examine a variety of other systems to define the mechanisms responsible for information storage at the synapse.

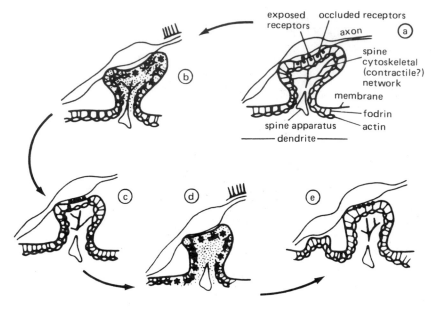

Figure 2.7
Proposed manner in which changed synaptic shape may be associated with long-term
potentiation. In this speculative series of events, the resting synapse, and postsynaptic
spine, are pictured in a. Impulse activity results in the influx of Ca^{++} into the postsynaptic spine, resulting in altered spine shape, presumably resulting from alterations in
the postsynaptic cytoskeleton. Alteration in shape results in strengthening of subsequent synaptic transmission. d and e depict even higher-frequency stimulation with
consequent alteration of postsynaptic spine shape. (From Lynch 1986)

Chapter 3

The Molecules: Transmitters as Prototypes

Characteristics of Cognitive Structures—Symbolic Function—Properties of Molecular Symbols—Transduction —Kinetics—Communicative Functions—Intracellular Cascades—Information, Syntax, and Semantics—Catecholamines, Tyrosine Hydroxylase, Fight-or-Flight—Enzyme Activation and Induction—Gene Regulation and the Environment—Experience and Behavior

Before discussing individual cognitive structures in detail, it may be useful to describe general features exhibited by these elements in the molecular and cellular domains. A relatively well-defined neural sub-system may serve as a prototype to indicate the locus occupied by communicative symbols in the economy of neural function and behavior.

The autonomic nervous system functions at the interface of environment and individual, translating external demands into appropriate physiological-vegetative and behavioral responses (figure 3.1). The system integrates environmental stimuli, internal metabolic state, and behavior, thereby serving a critical life function. The autonomic system has also been a traditional biological model, and biochemical regulatory mechanisms have been characterized in detail. In particular, the sympathetic division mediates the familiar fight-or-flight response to environmental threat or stress. Extensive study of this comparatively simple system has led to the biochemical picture described in chapter 2. A number of molecular species regulate function of the sympathetic nervous system. Certain threatening or stressful environmental stimuli elicit long-term sympathetic activation, and behavioral alteration, by altering the function of selected critical molecules. In turn, these molecules mediate the fight-or-flight reaction. In general terms, then, the molecules represent environmental stress and translate stress into components of the fight-or-flight behavioral-metabolic repertoire.

44   Chapter 3

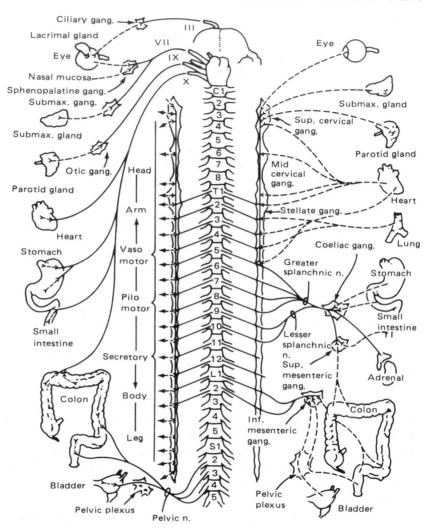

Figure 3.1
Schematic representation of the peripheral autonomic nervous system. The spinal cord and brain stem are pictured with the sympathetic ganglia and nerves on the right and the parasympathetic subdivision on the left. (After Harrison 1962)

We can now delineate a number of provisonal characteristics of cognitive molecular structures, based on initial consideration of the sympathetic system. The molecular elements:

1. Serve a semantic, **symbolic** function, representing external or internal reality.

2. **Communicate**, transmitting information among neuronal populations, aggregates, and ensembles, thereby forming biochemical circuits of information flow.

3. Govern moment-to-moment and long-term neural function, accessing the neuronal genome, regulating neuronal growth, and, more generally, dictating the **syntax** of communication and representation in the nervous system.

4. Constitute fundamental units in a more complex **combinatorial** system of higher order structures.

It will be useful to describe each of these characteristics and functions briefly, to place this approach in perspective and context, before discussing individual molecules in detail. How is symbolic function realized in the nervous system? Neural structures that are regulated by specific environmental stimuli, that change function in response to those stimuli, may **represent** those external stimuli in the nervous system.

Symbolic Function Is System Specific

Symbolic function is incorporated by certain molecules only in the context of specific neural systems in which the molecules are elaborated. For example, the same molecular symbol has very different "meanings" in sensory, somatic motor, or autonomic systems, which mediate different physiological repertoires. Thus, the "meaning" of a molecule is determined by regulating environmental events, function of the neural system regulated, and nature of the molecular function regulated. Symbolic function is conferred by specific environmental stimuli that regulate molecule state and function, physiological function of the relevant neural system, and function of the molecular structure in the economy of the specific neural system. Molecular semantics cannot be abstracted out of the neural system and nervous system. Molecules serve semantic functions only in the context of the nervous system and environment. Consequently, meaning, at the level of molecule, is conferred in multiple domains—the cellular, systems, organismic, and environmental levels. The information represented by a molecule is dependent on functions in virtually all other levels of the nervous system.

Although specific symbols regulate sympathetic function, it would be erroneous to assume that these particular molecules function at the nexus of stress and fight-or-flight throughout the nervous system. For example, the same molecules regulate function in other neural systems, including motor circuits governing movement and posture. Entirely different environmental stimuli regulate molecular function in these motor systems, and the molecules serve motor, not fight-or-flight, functions in these systems. In sum, the "meaning" of a molecular species is stimuli and system specific; semantics cannot be abstracted out of the context of neural subsystem. In this sense, the molecule has no "meaning" in the test tube, although molecular function may be preserved. This brief digression, trivial though it may seem, indicates the inadequacies of extreme reductionism, an approach of appealing simplicity.

Properties of Molecular Symbols

What should we want to know about symbolic function? What information is needed for symbol classification and for adequate characterization of symbol sets? The form and content of symbolic function are conferred by specific features that may be explicitly identified. These features are conveniently categorized by following the flow of information from environment to organism and neural system, and back to environment (figure 3.2).

The precise function of individual symbols derives from (1) regulatory environmental stimuli, (2) physicochemical characteristics of the particular molecule that confer function, (3) specific cellular and genomic properties that dictate the kinetics of regulation, (4) physiologic function of the neural subsystem in which the molecule is elaborated, (5) biochemical function of the molecule, and (6) role of the molecule in the complex biochemical-physiologic-behavioral web that defines syntactic function. A description of traits conferred by each category may help illustrate the potential spectrum and substance of symbolic functions.

The sympathetic nervous system continues to serve as a convenient example. Stressful stimuli regulate a number of functionally critical molecules in sympathetic neurons that govern fight-or-flight reactions. Consequently, in the context of the sympathetic system, these molecules that control function **represent** environmental stress and simultaneously contribute to the fight-or-flight physiologic-behavioral repertoire (figure 3.2). This simple example, moreover, indicates that environmental **stimuli possess structure** that allows construction of a **taxonomy**. For example, stressful stimuli may be classified as primary

Molecular Regulation

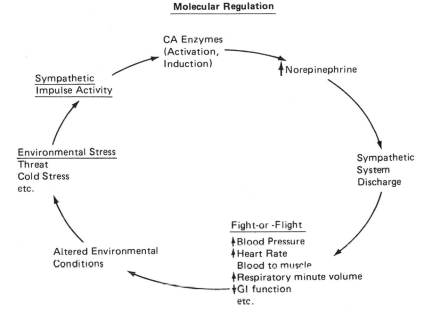

Figure 3.2
Molecular symbols and information flow—a very general scheme for the interaction of environmental stimuli, neuronal molecules, the flow of information, and resultant behavior.

sensory or secondary. Primary sensory consists of such types as cold stress, heat stress, and electric shock. Secondary may consist of immobilization stress or swimming stress, for example, depending on the experimental animal examined. It is apparent that a hierarchy of environmental stimuli may be constructed for any given neural symbol set. The precise relationship among elements of a stimulus set in regulating a symbol remains to be determined. In fact, the relationship may differ among individuals, species, genera, and others. Without belaboring the point, it is evident that environmental stimuli may be tentatively organized into a coherent schema based on symbols regulated. Indeed, classification of stimuli in terms of quantitative aspects of symbols regulated may represent an important contribution to understanding neural function in general and environment-neural relations in particular.

While the environment endows the regulated molecule with "meaning," the physical structure of the molecule, and the locus of the molecule in the structure of cell and system, determine the manner in which environmental stimulus is translated into neural function. For example, if the molecule happens to be an enzyme that synthesizes neurotransmitter, which communicates with other neurons, the activity of the enzyme is of critical importance. The activity of each individual molecule determines the rate of transmitter synthesis and the potential for communication and physiologic function. In turn, enzyme activity is determined by the structure of the enzyme molecule in three-dimensional space. Any alteration that changes molecule shape in space (conformation) may potentially alter activity and transmitter synthesis. In fact, many stimuli alter molecular structure, leading to a change in conformation and activity.

While molecules undergo a variety of reactions that alter structure, the specific reactions to which any given molecule is susceptible are determined by molecular structure. For example, particular structures allow phosphorylation, a common mode of alteration in biologic systems (for review, see Nestler and Greengard 1984). Phosphorylation, or the addition of phosphate groups to a molecule, changes conformation and activity (figure 3.3). Since the chemical reactions for phosphorylation and dephosphorylation exhibit characteristic kinetics, the temporal properties of this type of environmental regulation are defined, to a significant degree, by the structure of the actual molecular symbols regulated. Other (posttranslational) mechanisms that alter structure and function include such chemical reactions as amidation, methylation, and glycosylation.

The alteration of structure of molecules already present in the cell falls into a broad category termed posttranslational processing (the processing of gene products that have already been translated into cellular proteins, such as enzymes). Other modes of environmental regulation consist of alteration of the number of molecules in the cell, not simply alteration of those already present. While altered molecule number may occur through a variety of mechanisms, one prominent process involves altered synthesis from the gene. Indeed, many stimuli alter the synthesis of functionally important gene products, thereby altering the number of molecules in the cell. To a first approximation, the number of molecules of any type represents a balance between synthesis and all those processes leading to decay. Consequently a change in synthetic rate is associated with a marked change in the level of any molecular species in the cell.

In fact, environmental stimuli frequently alter the readout of functionally important genes (synthesis from the gene). The actual time course of altered synthesis, altered levels of gene product, and resultant altered function depends on the characteristics of the particular gene affected and the metabolic machinery of the specific cell (neuron) type. Consequently the temporal profile of changed cell and system

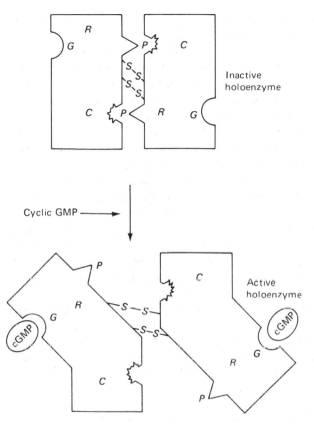

Figure 3.3
Phosphorylation alters molecular conformation (three dimensional shape). Schematic representation of a particular enzyme in which cyclic GMP (cGMP) phosphorylates the molecule, resulting in a change in shape. The inactive, baseline enzyme is pictured above, and the effect of cyclic GMP binding on molecular conformation is pictured below. The binding of cGMP converts the inactive enzyme to a biologically active molecule. (From Nestler and Greengard 1984)

function, whether transient or quasi-permanent, is dependent on biologic organization. While stimuli trigger biologic mechanism, the form and content of neural change are dictated by biology, not environment. The rules of biology determine the transformational functions that convert environmental to neural information.

The kinetics, the computational aspects of environmental regulation and symbolic function, represent a summation of the processes described—whether posttranslational or genomic. The computations performed by neurons and systems are composed of these individual regulatory operations. Examination of a prototypical instance of environmentally regulated, increased gene readout may identify some of the variables involved and some of the more important parameters. In figure 3.4 a specific stimulus, such as a stress, increases the readout of a gene encoding a neurotransmitter. The number of transmitter molecules in the neural subsystem increases, with augmented function. The temporal profile of altered behavior results from the profile of altered biochemical regulation. Several simple parameters characterize the biological response and give the resultant behavior its form. Initial behavioral change depends on the **lag** between stimulus and increased transmitter elaboration. The **doubling time** of the response represents the time required for molecule number to increase twofold from initial baseline levels and reflects the new **rate constant** for synthesis (balanced against the process of ongoing degradation). The doubling time and synthesis rate constant reflect properties of individual genes and differ for different genes. In addition, the magnitude of increase in molecule number is also dependent on the specific gene stimulated and the neuron or cell type involved. Finally, in this simplified example, the duration of the response, a function of the half-time of decay (apparent half-life), is determined by genomic and cellular organization dictating rates of degradation of the molecular species. Consequently different gene products exhibit different kinetics of regulation and mediate different behavioral time courses, based on internal, biological imperatives. At present the specifics of organization for any given product are defined empirically.

These introductory remarks indicate that symbols are manipulated according to the rules of internal cell biology while simultaneously representing external, extracellular stimuli. Moreover, meaning is conferred by physiologic function of the subsystem to which the symbol is localized, in addition to the relevant environmental stimuli, and rules of cellular and molecular biology.

The syntactic properties of a symbol, or symbol set, are defined by many of the same organizational features that are central to semantic function. Organization of genome, cell or neuronal type, and specific

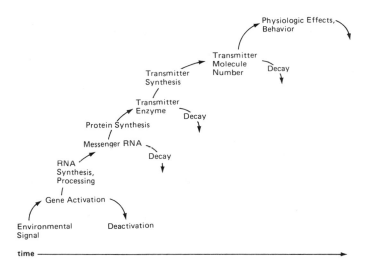

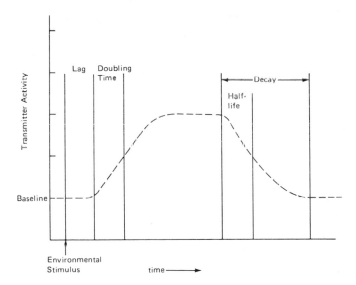

Figure 3.4
(a) Environmental regulatory cascade: A simplified scheme of molecular turnover. A general schematic representation of the manner in which environmental stimuli alter physiology and behavior through a sequence of molecular transformations. Note that each particular element depicted turns over with characteristic kinetics or time constants.
(b) Schematic representation of the basic aspects of the kinetics of transmitter regulation. Note that alteration of transmitter status by the environment may be defined according to characteristic stages. The temporal characteristics of the regulation of any individual transmitter are unique to that transmitter system.

neural subsystem defines functional relations of symbols. Physico-chemical structure of the molecular symbol defines its biochemical role in the economy of cell and system, whether enzymatic, neurotrans-mission, growth promoting, and/or hormonal. Further, symbols com-monly elicit multiple short- and long-term effects simultaneously. For example, transmitters mediate millisecond-to-millisecond communi-cation among neurons while regulating long-term functions such as enzyme induction, synapse growth, and nerve process growth. On the other hand, the same symbol, molecular species may respond to a family of stimuli. Consequently symbols integrate information from multiple external stimuli and transduce this information into multiple biologic responses (figure 3.2). Detailed aspects of syntactic function are discussed individually as each specific symbol is examined.

Communicative Functions

Although traditional teaching maintained that communication in the nervous system consisted entirely of millisecond-to-millisecond elec-trochemical transmission, recent discoveries indicate that this view is far too restrictive. Communication and its sequelae are mediated by diverse classes of signal operating over a range of time courses and governing manifold cell and system functions. In fact, increasing ev-idence indicates that orthodox distinctions among transmitters, growth factors, trophic factors (survival factors), and hormones, for example, are routinely violated. For instance, many transmitters si-multaneously mediate rapid, electrical communication, foster neuron survival and consequent pathway formation, elicit synaptic change with enhanced circuit function, and trigger biochemical changes that amplify subsequent signal transmission (for examples, see Denis-Donini 1989; Mudge 1989; Pincus et al. 1990). Conversely, multiple signal classes converge to regulate such individual functions as rapid communication, survival, and growth.

Nevertheless, different general categories of communicative (or con-nectional) agents may be delineated, based on routes of delivery. For example, transmitters tend to operate through point-to-point com-munication, while hormones affect distant targets. On the other hand, growth factors function through autocrine (same cell), paracrine (prox-imate cells), and endocrine (remote cells) modes. However, all these signal molecules contribute to communication itself or to the regula-tion of connection strength.

While different signal classes, and different molecules within a class, occupy different functional loci, specific molecules may be localized to identifiable nodes within a functional matrix (figure 3.2). The particular locus occupied by a signal dictates its role in the syntax of function of any specific neural subsystem. An idealized, hypothetical example is depicted in figure 3.2. The transmitter elicits all physiological effects by binding to a specific family of receptors. However, the consequences of receptor binding are manifold and heterogeneous. Binding evokes rapid changes in the conductance of specific ion channels, leading to altered membrane voltage and action potentials over milliseconds. Impulse activity evokes a variety of downstream physiological and behavioral responses, based on the activation of multiple neural and effector pathways. The rapid electrogenic effects represent traditional transmitter function. In addition, receptor binding activates other biochemical-physiological cascades, with intermediate- and long-term consequences. For example, altered membrane voltage, due to transmitter action, allows Ca^{++} influx through voltage-gated channels. Ca^{++}, in turn, acts as an intracellular messenger, regulating a variety of biochemical processes. Ca^{++} activates a group of proteolytic enzymes that may remodel the synapse and synaptic spine, resulting in enhanced subsequent transmission (for example, see Lynch 1986). Ca^{++} also activates enzymes that phosphorylate synaptic proteins mediating transmission, thereby altering functional connectivity through additional mechanisms (for review, see Nestler and Greengard 1984). Although Ca^{++} exhibits a variety of other actions, these few examples illustrate the nature of the cascade.

Receptor binding activates additional intracellular messenger pathways, resulting in protean responses (figure 3.5). Activation of the enzyme adenylyl cyclase results in the hydrolysis of ATP (adenosine triphosphate) to form cyclic AMP (adenosine monophosphate). Consequently a variety of functionally critical proteins are phosphorylated, leading to altered synaptic transmission, altered synthesis and release of postsynaptic transmitter, and altered readout of genes coding for entirely different transmitters. Receptor activation of the phosphorylation cascade radically alters the efficacy of specific neural circuits and even changes the nature of circuits by altering the mix of transmitters elaborated.

Activation of yet another intracellular biochemical network results in complementary responses. The phosphotidylinositol cascade, which elaborates intracellular signal phospholipids, regulates a variety of enzyme activities and governs the transcription of many critical genes concerned with intercellular communication. Receptor binding activates portions of this pathway, resulting in an additional array of responses that also changes subsequent transmission.

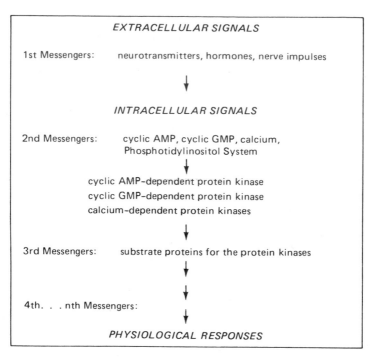

EXTRACELLULAR SIGNALS

1st Messengers: neurotransmitters, hormones, nerve impulses

INTRACELLULAR SIGNALS

2nd Messengers: cyclic AMP, cyclic GMP, calcium,
Phosphotidylinositol System

cyclic AMP-dependent protein kinase
cyclic GMP-dependent protein kinase
calcium-dependent protein kinases

3rd Messengers: substrate proteins for the protein kinases

4th. . . nth Messengers:

PHYSIOLOGICAL RESPONSES

Figure 3.5
Examples of signal cascades. Extracellular signals are converted to intracellular information through a series of transduction processes involving the molecular messengers depicted. (After Nestler and Greengard 1984)

Finally, the Ca^{++}, phosphorylation, and phospholipid cascades are mutually regulatory: information flows from one pathway to the other, resulting in complex excitatory and inhibitory interactions.

The hypothetical transmitter is regulated by specific environmental stimuli. Consequently specific and selective environmental stimuli gain access to the intracellular processes that constitute the substance of information processing in the nervous system. Moreover, the communicative molecule functions symbolically, selectively transducing specific environmental stimuli into specific neural information. In turn, that information is not indifferent. The information comprises the operational rules and the very operation of the nervous system. The information is the syntax of the system. Syntax and semantics are one in the same in the nervous system.

With this general introduction, specific examples of symbolic function may be fruitfully examined. Initially the well-defined, relatively simple autonomic nervous system may continue to serve as the paradigm.

Communicative Symbols and Transducer Molecules

Certain molecules within the nervous system are capable of acting as transducers, converting one form of information into another. Further, this transduction process may change communication among neurons. It may be particularly illustrative to choose one example and describe the processes, pointing out implications for neural function as we proceed.

Neurotransmitters, the chemical molecular signals sent from one neuron to another, are quintessential communicative symbols in the nervous system. Although their communicative functions have long been apparent, their symbolic functions have not been recognized. Yet these molecular signals are known to change in highly specific ways in response to environmental events. And alteration of transmitter function markedly changes communication among neurons. How can we relate environmental change, transmitter change, change in neural state, and change in neural function? To approach these issues, we examine catecholamines, some of the most widely studied transmitters. The catecholamines, including dopamine, norepinephrine, and epinephrine, mediate peripheral and central functions, from the vegetative to the cognitive. A variety of molecules can alter catecholamine function, but we will focus on a single regulatory molecule, tyrosine hydroxylase (TH), since it exemplifies a number of transduction mechanisms. These processes are central to symbolic and communicative function.

TH is the rate-limiting enzyme in catecholamine biosynthesis; the activity of this enzyme determines the rate of synthesis of these transmitters (figure 2.3; Levitt et al. 1965). Consequently TH catalytic activity regulates transmitter synthesis in the sympathoadrenal axis peripherally and in central aminergic nuclei in the brain. Ongoing synthesis of catecholamines is particularly important since it is the newly synthesized pool of transmitter that is preferentially released upon stimulation (for review, see Molinoff and Axelrod 1971). How does TH alter catecholamine biosynthesis? A variety of complex molecular processes alter TH activity and hence catecholamine biosynthesis; all of the known processes ultimately triggered by environmental stimuli (external to the neuron or organism). For example, stressful stimuli increase TH activity (for example, see Thoenen et al. 1969), leading to increased amine synthesis and mobilization for the fight-or-flight response. Consequently TH is a typical transducer molecule.

As an example, increased neuronal impulse frequency increases TH and results in elevation of catecholamine biosynthesis. In the sympathetic system, increased impulse activity, in turn, is elicited by stressful environmental stimuli. Consequently TH may be regarded as a neural molecule that transduces environmental events into altered neurotransmitter synthesis and sympathetic neuron function.

What molecular mechanisms underlie changes in TH activity? There are fundamentally two ways in which TH activity may increase: the activity of each molecule may rise without a change in the total number of molecules per cell, or the actual number of TH molecules may increase, resulting in a rise in total TH activity in the neuron (figure 3.4; for example, see Zigmond et al. 1989 for discussion). Available evidence suggests that both of these generic mechanisms do occur physiologically with increased impulse activity.

Enzyme Activation

TH is subject to feedback inhibition by the transmitter products dopamine and norepinephrine (figure 2.3). That is, these transmitter products actually decrease the (catalytic) activity of each TH molecule, thereby reducing the synthesis of L-DOPA from tyrosine. Consequently the biosynthesis of dopamine, norepinephrine, and epinephrine is reduced (figure 2.3). Increased impulse activity, however, decreases the concentration of the feedback inhibitors in the neuronal cytoplasm, leading to a short-term increase in TH activity and catecholamine biosynthesis over seconds to minutes. This disinhibition of TH has the net effect of increasing the efficiency of each functional (catalytic) site on existent TH molecules without changing total TH molecule number.

To summarize, using the sympathetic system as a model, stress increases neuron impulse activity, reducing concentrations of the feedback inhibitors dopamine and norepinephrine, leading to increased TH activity and catecholamine transmitter biosynthesis. Clearly this is one instance of an enzyme transducing environmental stimuli into altered function in the nervous system. Other mechanisms, presumably triggered by increased neuronal impulse activity, may also increase the catalytic activity of each TH molecule. Using adrenomedullary catecholaminergic cells as models, recent work has demonstrated that stimulation with acetylcholine, the natural presynaptic transmitter, or depolarization itself (with veratridine) also increases the activity of TH, with a consequent rise in catecholamine biosynthesis (Waymire et al. 1988). In this instance, however, the critical molecular events appear to involve phosphorylation of the TH molecule by cyclic AMP with a consequent rise in TH catalytic activity. This effect occurs within 2 minutes and lasts approximately 30 minutes. Although relatively short term as well, this effect distinctly outlasts the inciting stimulus. This, then, is the first concrete example in which environmental change elicits a molecular alteration that persists and that changes cellular function.

The implied, but still somewhat speculative, sequence of events would involve (1) presynaptic release of acetylcholine, (2) cholinergic depolarization of the adrenomedullary cells, (3) phosphorylation of TH through as yet undefined mechanisms, (4) consequent TH activation and (5) increased catecholamine biosynthesis. The entire sequence of molecular events is triggered by environmental stress and results in the release of catecholamines from the adrenal, with well-described physiologic and behavioral consequences.

How might phosphorylation increase TH activity? Potentially phosphorylation at multiple sites in the molecule may alter the tertiary structure (shape and orientation in three-dimensional space) of the TH enzyme protein, leading to either enhanced efficiency of catalytic sites or exposure of additional catalytic sites (for example, see figure 3.3). Either event would increase catecholamine transmitter biosynthesis without changing the number of TH molecules in the cell.

Enzyme Induction

We have considered the first type of mechanism by which TH activity can increase: increased efficiency of each molecule that is already present. The second mechanism involves an entirely different process: increased activity consequent to an increase in the number of molecules. That is, environmental stimuli may increase TH activity in the long term by increasing the number of TH molecules, a process known as enzyme induction (Mueller et al. 1969; Thoenen et al. 1969). Stressful stimuli, such as swimming stress, cold stress and drugs that interfere with sympathetic function, increase sympathoadrenal impulse flow. Increased release of presynaptic acetylcholine, postsynaptic depolarization, and attendant transmembrane sodium ion influx result in an increase in the number of TH molecules in the neuron. Catecholamine synthesis rises accordingly.

In principle, the elevation of TH molecule number could be due to either an increased rate of synthesis of enzyme molecules or a decreased rate of degradation (figure 3.4). The balance of any molecular species in a cell is due to all of the events leading to synthesis and events causing degradation. Several lines of evidence suggest that the induction of TH is indeed due to elevated synthesis of the enzyme. Identification of specific mechanisms is critical for understanding how the nervous system translates environmental events into neural language.

Induction of TH in sympathetic neurons by increased impulse activity is blocked by inhibitors of protein and RNA synthesis (Mueller et al. 1969), indirectly suggesting that elevated synthesis may be critical. More recently experimental evidence indicates that increased nerve firing also elevates the mRNA (messenger RNA) coding for the TH protein (Black et al. 1985; Mallet et al. 1983). Importantly, denervation of these neurons, which prevents the reception of increased impulses and TH induction, also prevents the increase in TH mRNA. These results, viewed with those already cited, suggest that a sequence of events involving (1) environmental stress, (2) increased nerve impulse activity, (3) increased transmembrane sodium ion influx, (4) increased transcription of TH mRNA from DNA, and (5) increased synthesis of TH protein underlie induction of TH (for example, see figure 3.4).

Stated somewhat differently, it appears that environmental events may alter gene readout by altering nerve impulse activity. In turn, alteration of gene readout changes neural and behavioral function. This is not a particularly modest claim. Experience alters the function of neurons at the most fundamental level, the genome. How long do these neuronal changes last?

The kinetics of TH induction are particularly intriguing since brief environmental events are transduced into long-term neuronal changes. Environmental stress and increased sympathoadrenal impulse activity evoke a two- to three-fold increase in TH within two days and enzyme remains elevated for at least three days after increased impulse activity has ceased. In fact, direct nerve electrical stimulation for 30 to 90 minutes increases enzyme molecule number for at least three days (see Zigmond 1989 for review). Consequently a brief environmental stimulus is transduced into a long-term neuronal molecular change, providing striking **temporal amplification** by the nervous system.

The temporal amplification exhibited by TH displays a number of properties with notable implications for mind-brain molecules. For example, repetitive stimuli cause a far greater induction of TH than does a single stimulus. In one group of experiments, rats were treated with the pharmacologic agent reserpine, which mimics environmental stress by increasing sympathetic impulse activity. A single injection evoked a 2.5-fold rise in TH in three days. In striking contrast, repeated daily injections elicited a five-fold rise after five days (Mueller et al. 1969).

These observations were paralleled by direct electrical stimulation of the preganglionic sympathetic nerves. Stimulation at 10 (Hz) for only 10 minutes increased enzyme activity by 25 percent three days later, while excitation for 60 minutes elevated TH activity by 73 percent (Zigmond and Chalazonitis 1979; Zigmond 1980b). In summary, repetition and increased stimulus duration increase the magnitude of TH induction, as might be expected for a communicative symbol involved in memory. Certainly the kinetics of TH induction are intriguing, suggesting that functionally important transmitter regulatory molecules can store environmental information for relatively prolonged periods of time. How long?

To approach this important question, it is necessary to characterize the decrease in TH subsequent to induction. This has already been partially accomplished. Subsequent to induction, the half-time of decay is approximately two days, and normal basal levels of enzyme are approximated one week after initial stimulation (Thoenen et al. 1970). The decrease in TH is regulated, presumably, by specific neuronal proteolytic degrading enzymes, which metabolize TH itself.

To summarize, a single example, TH, illustrates some of the molecular mechanisms the nervous system uses to transduce environmental events into functionally significant neural language. The particular characteristics of the functions will vary naturally from molecule to molecule, each with its particular biologic function, kinetic characteristics, stimuli to which it is responsive, and so forth. TH simply served as a convenient model to illustrate a number of salient points.

Nevertheless, the molecular mechanisms examined are of critical import for the organism. TH, as a critical regulator of the sympathoadrenal axis, plays a pivotal role in the well-known fight-or-flight reaction. This behavioral-emotional repertoire is elicited by environmental stress and depends on sympathoadrenal activation, in which TH is of central importance. The repertoire includes pupillary dilation, piloerection, increased cardiac output, general shunting of blood toward striated muscle, increased respiratory minute volume, contraction of vesicle and anal sphincters, and reduced peristalsis—reactions associated with mobilization for emergency. Consequently increased TH activity is a functionally critical component in the transduction of environmental stress into activation of a specific neural system with defined behavioral sequelae.

Questions may be raised concerning the specificity of the environmental stimulus and the evoked neural response. If a variety of environmental stressful situations evoke similar flight-or-fight reactions, can this be relevant to brain function that exhibits such extraordinary specificities? This understandable question misses the point that physiologic responses, evoked by an aggregate of molecular interactions, are system specific. The sympathetic system mediates the foregoing physiologic responses—not speech, not vision, not olfaction. Specificity of physiologic response resides in the system. The response is mediated and constrained by the communicative symbolic molecules that govern function of the system. Although the examples thus far have been drawn from the periphery, in the next chapter we examine direct relevance of the same molecular mechanisms to brain function.

The central point, however, bears restatement: essential functions of the nervous system are performed in the molecular domain. Specific communicative symbolic molecules convert environmental or internal information into altered neural function and behavior.

Can we now use TH, as an example, to indicate how molecular processes interact with other symbol sets? We examine this explicitly in the following chapter.

Chapter 4

From Molecule to Brain Function and Behavior

Tyrosine Hydroxylase, Locus Coeruleus, and Attention—A Role in Anxiety?—Topography and Transport—Substantia Nigra and Motor Behavior—Form and Content in Behavior—Some Characteristics of Memory

In the previous chapter, we used TH as a prototypical transducer molecule to examine function in the relatively simple peripheral nervous system. Surprisingly, perhaps, it was possible to discern a causal relationship between TH, a communicative molecular symbol, and a behavioral complex, the fight-or-flight reaction. In principle, then, the apparently vast gulf between molecule and behavior can be bridged, at least in the comparatively straightforward periphery. Is this approach applicable to the brain? Alternatively, is brain function so complex that examination of a single molecule will prove unrevealing?

It may be helpful to pose some central questions at the outset. How do we begin to understand such apparent brain states as alertness, attention, vigilance, and anxiety in terms of molecular function? That question seems to be all but unapproachable at present. Let us consider another set of brain functions initially. Can we comprehend how the brain coordinates bodily movement by examining molecular function? A slight change of perspective may be helpful. We can frame a more general question in familiar terms. How does the brain receive, transduce, encode, store, and transmit information? Do any central processes resemble those in the periphery? Are similar molecular processes involved?

In fact, we can usefully begin discussions by considering those systems in the brain that use TH. As we shall see, examination of the role of TH in the economy of brain function will lead to insights even more startling than those attained in the periphery. However, at the outset, I must stress that we are focusing on a single molecule in a system that uses multitudinous molecules and aggregates of molecules. My goal is certainly not to explain all of the foregoing brain functions in terms of a single molecular species. Rather, I hope to use a now-familiar prototype to illustrate the principles of moving from molecule to brain state to behavior and mental function. If we can begin to approach this relatively modest goal, then the more formidable task of relating multiple molecules to a variety of functions is, in theory, attainable. (In the course of employing TH as a prototype, readers may learn a bit more about a particular subject than they care to know. However, the knowledge, like most other coins of the realm, is transferable and purchases insights in many different spheres of the mind-brain world.)

For illustrative purposes, we initially examine the issues of alertness, attention, vigilance, and anxiety in terms of a specific brain subsystem and its molecular mechanisms.

The locus coeruleus is a bilateral group of several thousand neurons in the brain stem that projects throughout the neuraxis (Swanson and Hartman 1975; Nygren and Olson 1977; for review, see Moore and Bloom 1979). Locus cells innervate the cerebral cortex rostrally and cerebellar Purkinje cells and cortex superiorly and also project inferiorly to innervate neurons within the spinal cord (figure 4.1). Through

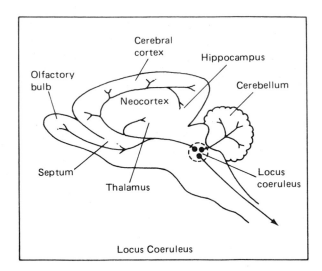

Figure 4.1
Schematic representation of the locus coeruleus. The locus coeruleus is depicted as a group of cell bodies lying in the rostral pons of the brain stem. Fibers project rostrally to the telencephalon, including the neocortex, superiorly to the cerebellum and inferiorly to the spinal cord. (From Kuffler et al. 1984)

this remarkable anatomical arrangement, the locus is in a position to influence neurons at virtually all levels of the CNS.

The classic work of Bloom and colleagues suggests that the locus sets levels of vigilance or alertness in arrays of central neurons (for example, see Aston-Jones and Bloom 1981a, 1981b). The locus, which is activated by multimodal somatosensory stimuli, appears to bias central neurons globally, orienting the CNS to either environmental or internal demands. For example, spontaneous discharge of locus neurons correlates with stages of the sleep-wake cycle, exhibiting rates that vary directly with the level of vigilance in behaving rats. Spontaneous and sensory-evoked activity is tonically reduced during sleep, grooming, and feeding but is phasically augmented with interruption of such behaviors. Based on these and analogous observations, Bloom and coworkers propose that environmental stimuli elicit the release of locus norepinephrine that simultaneously enhances activity of target brain systems engaged by environmental sensory stimuli while suppressing systems involved in tonic vegetative (internal) functions. The net effect is to increase vigilance and those phasic brain functions that adapt the organism to changing environmental demands. In summary, low levels of locus activity may bias target systems that govern vegetative functions, whereas abrupt increases in activity elicited by quasi-emergent environmental demands enhance signal-to-noise, and therefore activity, in systems mediating adaptation to external events. Consequently the locus may facilitate transitions between behavioral states (Aston-Jones and Bloom 1981a, 1981b).

Returning to one of our initial questions, the locus system appears to play a key role in eliciting alertness, attention, and vigilance; these states are favored by the release of norepinephrine from appropriate locus terminals. With this background, we are now in a position to begin analyzing locus function, and attendant attention and vigilance, in terms of molecular mechanism. Indeed, can we begin to understand these brain and behavioral states by examining communicative molecular symbols? Our discussions concerning molecular function in the peripheral nervous system are directly relevant to analysis of brain processes for several reasons. The locus, as a noradrenergic nucleus, uses precisely the same biosynthetic pathway as sympathetics to elaborate norepinephrine (for review, see Moore and Bloom 1979). TH molecules in locus and sympathetics appear to be identical structurally, indicating that a number of control mechanisms are operative in brain as in periphery (for review, see Zigmond et al. 1989). For example, inhibition and activation of the enzyme occur in locus just as in sympathetics. Similarly cellular control mechanisms, including enzyme induction, so important for regulation in sympathetics, also occur in the locus (Zigmond et al. 1974; Black 1975; Zigmond 1979). Simply stated, the same rules that govern function of this molecular symbol in sympathetics also govern function in the locus. To summarize, TH in the locus is subject to feedback inhibition by reaction products, activation through phosphorylation, and enzyme induction, an increase in the number of enzyme molecules.

How can we relate these molecular processes to attention, alertness, and vigilance? Will an understanding of molecular mechanism in the locus provide deeper insights into the phenomena of attention and vigilance? Will formerly unrecognized features of these mental states become apparent? We begin by considering the acute effects of activating the locus. Abrupt, short-term increases in environmental somatosensory stimuli, resulting in increased locus discharge, acutely disinhibit and activate TH in locus terminals. Elevated locus terminal release of norepinephrine (NE), associated with reduced cytoplasmic concentrations of the dopamine and norepinephrine feedback inhibitors, disinhibits TH, resulting in elevated NE synthesis. Consequently augmented NE is available for release and increased interaction with target receptors. As a result of these acute effects, the animal becomes alert and attentive. TH obviously plays a critical role in this biochemical-behavioral cascade since it is rate limiting in the synthesis of NE, the transmitter that mediates arousal. In addition to this obvious role, TH functions symbolically to link environment to behavioral state.

The same mechanisms that are so important in the generation of the flight-or-fight reaction in the periphery are equally critical in the generation of attention and alertness in the coeruleal system. Environmental somatosensory stimulation enhances locus discharge, leading to TH activation through phosphorylation at multiple sites (as in the adrenomedullary cells). Moreover, we already know, from discussions of the peripheral nervous system, that stimuli lasting seconds to minutes result in phosphorylation activation lasting half an hour. That is, the detailed kinetics described in the previous chapter suggest that a temporally circumscribed stimulus results in neural activation lasting 30 minutes. Consequently environmental stimuli are **temporally amplified** resulting in relatively long-lasting TH changes that globally increase CNS vigilance for half an hour.

Knowledge of the kinetics of TH activation allows us to move from the molecular to synaptic, systems, and behavioral domains and draw some surprising conclusions. On the basis of enzyme activation, one would predict that sensory stimuli lasting seconds potentially prepare the locus for unanticipated, future events over the subsequent half-hour. The TH communicative symbol therefore serves a behavioral anticipatory function. In essence, the molecular architecture of the locus system is so constructed that a single threatening event elicits changes designed to anticipate another, immediate threat. Threat (or stress) simultaneously alerts acutely and readies the organism for repeated threat in the near future. One can easily understand the potential survival value of such a molecular-neural arrangement. It should be emphasized that these behavioral insights, and implicit constraints, derive entirely from our understanding of molecular mechanism. (But surely a multitude of biochemical changes transpire in the stress response that results in vigilance. Indeed there must be. TH is merely a prototype for the kind of molecular mechanism that explains and elucidates the nature of attention and alertness. We shall turn to other molecules, other symbols, and other mechanisms as we proceed).

Consideration of TH induction in the present context leads to a number of startling conclusions. Agents that increase impulse flow in the periphery also induce TH in the locus. To recap, TH induction consists of an increase in the number of enzyme molecules. Enzyme induction occurs in locus perikarya in the pons, and the increased enzyme is subsequently transported distally to target terminals (Black 1975; Zigmond 1978), resulting in elevated synthesis of NE. The time course of these effects is of extreme interest. After drug treatment, TH reaches peak activity in 4 days in locus perikarya, in 8 days in the proximate cerebellum, but only after 12 days in the distant frontal cortex (Black 1975; figure 4.2). Thus, the frontal cortex in particular, and the neocortex in general, are subjected to delayed and prolonged elevation of TH activity, with enhanced NE synthesis. Consequently the cortical substrates of increased vigilance and alertness persist long after the exciting environmental stimulus is gone. Conversely cortical systems subserving vegetative functions may remain suppressed for prolonged periods.

It may be useful to consider the implications of these observations. A brief environmental stimulus sets in motion a series of events that results in long-term changes, lasting weeks in locus cortical terminals. On the basis of TH induction and the geometry of proximo-distal axonal transport, the brain remains poised for attention and vigilance for **weeks**. Is this memory? If so, it certainly is an unconventional form. We usually think of memory for information or even for procedures such as bike riding or piano playing. However, the present "memory" is that of a brain state. This phenomenon does have many of the characteristics of traditional memory, however. For example, it is subject to rehearsal effects and does decay. The decay (see figure 3.4), which we may term forgetting, can be quantitatively described in terms of the progressive fall in TH activity in cortical terminals.

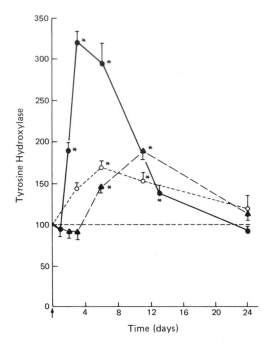

Figure 4.2
Time course of the increase in TH activity in locus coeruleus (closed circles), cerebellum
(open circles), and frontal cortex (closed triangles) after reserpine treatment (arrow).
Rats were treated with reserpine at time 0 or with saline. At varying times after injection,
groups of six control and six reserpine-treated animals were killed, and enzyme activity
was assayed in the indicated areas. Results are expressed as percentage of respective
controls plus or minus SEM (vertical bars).
** Differs from respective control at $p < 0.001$. (From Black 1975)

Clearly we may have to alter our conception of memory, based on elementary considerations of molecular mechanism and cell biology in the brain. At the very least, TH appears to function as a communicative symbol—a molecule that receives, encodes, stores, and transmits information over time.

While the arousal-vigilance complex may represent a long-term adaptive response to environmental stimulation, the potential for maladaptation cannot be excluded out of hand. Extensive studies by Redmond and colleagues in primates indicate that electrical stimulation of the locus results in behavioral repertoires and physiologic changes characteristic of "fear" and "anxiety" (Redmond et al. 1976, 1979; but also see Mason and Fibiger 1979). Pharmacologic antagonists which prevent discharge, inhibit these responses. Moreover, pharmacologic stimulation of the locus with piperoxane (an alpha-adrenergic antagonist) elicits similar effects. Further, in related observations, Aghajanian and colleagues have found that the locus, which receives innervation from multiple pain pathways, exhibits sustained discharge in response to repeated presentation of noxious stimuli (Cedarbaum and Aghajanian, 1976).

Redmond has related these results to a role of the locus in anxiety states. Locus stimulation and discharge, in this view, are associated with the anxiety attendant to noxious stimulation, arousal, and increased vigilance. Indeed, the locus does innervate targets responsible for physiological reactions associated with pain and fear. What is the potential role of the TH molecular symbol in this complex behavioral-experimental syndrome?

Stimulation of the locus by somatosensory input, including noxious stimuli, results in rapid activation and disinhibition of TH in all locus terminals, with consequent increases in NE synthesis in terminals throughout the nervous system. **However, the resulting enzyme induction will have very different effects in different terminals.** In particular the distant cerebrocortical terminals—those associated with vigilance, arousal, and perhaps anxiety—will be subjected to delayed and prolonged elevation of TH and NE biosynthesis (see figure 4.2). The stage will be set for the manifestation and experience of delayed anxiety consequent to sensory stimulation. Thus, TH may play a role in "normal" anxiety attendant to locus stimulation by environmental events.

Recent work, moreover, has indicated that many of the cortical areas that are innervated by the locus in turn innervate the locus through feedback pathways. In addition, as I have already mentioned, multiple pain pathways innervate the locus. In principle, then, endogenous activity, whether normal or abnormal, can theoretically activate locus neurons. One consequence of such increased discharge would be maintained, elevated TH levels in the cortex, with the potential for anxiety syndromes. Anxiety may be generated, consequently, from primarily external or internal events.

We now return to the implications of TH decay in the cortex with time. After reaching peak activity 12 days subsequent to stimulation, TH gradually decreases, approximating basal levels by 24 days (figure 4.2). Consequently it is possible to estimate that the increased potential for anxiety reactions after an exciting stimulus lasts approximately two weeks, based on our knowledge of the TH time course in cortical terminals. Although such estimates are speculative, they serve to illustrate how knowledge of underlying molecular processes can inform inquiries into behavioral states. The temporal profile of a behavioral or mental state is intimately related to the function of the molecular symbols involved. The symbols shape a mental state, accounting for many of its characteristics, and in fact are part and parcel of the state itself.

It is apparent that I have focused on TH exclusively in our approach to an extremely complicated system, the locus coeruleus, and extremely complex behavioral repertoires. My goal has been to indicate how the behavior of a single molecular species may affect a relatively well-defined neural system and psychologic function. I certainly do not intend to attribute all locus actions to a single molecular type. Rather, TH has simply served as a convenient prototype. Multiple mind-brain molecules will follow.

Molecular Symbols and the Behavior-Motor Interface

Employing a moderate degree of tunnel vision, we have focused on the single molecule TH to begin defining relationships among multiple functions in the mind-brain system. Even limiting our focus, however, we have been able to explore the role of TH in very different neural systems and behavioral repertoires: TH participates in the sympathoadrenal fight-or-flight reactions and in the locus coeruleus arousal-vigilance complex. In the locus, moreover, the potential role of TH in the pathogenesis of anxiety was described. A final case study, focusing on human disease, complements examples already discussed and emphasizes the practical implications of our inquiry.

Parkinson's disease, or paralysis agitans, has cursed human existence through the ages; descriptions extend back to antiquity. Typically the affected individual suffers from slowed movements (bradykinesia), difficulty initiating movements, a masklike face, muscle rigidity, stooped gait, and a slow (4–6 per second) tremor. Some patients are subject to dementia. The ongoing solution of this clinical problem represents one of the happiest basic science-clinical collaborative efforts in neurology. It also typifies the relationship between molecules and behavior. In the mid-1950s Arvid Carlsson, a Swedish scientist, continued his investigations of the neurochemistry of the substantia nigra and its connections to the basal ganglia (figure 4.3). He strongly suspected that dopamine might be involved in nigrostriatal neurotransmission (for example, see Carlsson et al. 1958). To pursue his experiments, he used the drug reserpine, an agent known to deplete monoamines throughout the body. Rats injected with the agent exhibited a curious syndrome: they were hypokinetic, nearly motionless, assumed a humped-back, splay-footed posture, and suffered from a coarse, whole body tremor. Carlsson was struck by the resemblance to human Parkinson's patients. After measuring dopamine in the nigrostriatal system and noting profound depletion, he made the remarkable suggestion that decreased nigrostriatal dopamine might play a role in the pathogenesis of human Parkinson's disease.

Virtually simultaneously Oleh Hornykiewicz, an Austrian neuropathologist working in Canada, assayed dopamine in the brains of people succumbing during the course of Parkinson's disease (Ehringer and Hornykiewicz 1960; Birkmayer and Hornykiewicz 1961). He noted a striking decrease in the amine in the basal ganglia, supporting the

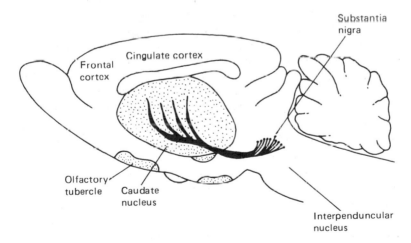

Figure 4.3
The nigrostriatal system. Nigrostriatal neurons are depicted projecting to the caudate nucleus of the striatum. The nigrostriatal system plays a critical role in the regulation of motor behavior and degenerates in Parkinson's disease. (After Cooper et al. 1982)

contention that dopamine deficiency was associated with this long-mysterious movement disorder.

George Cotzias, a clinician studying and caring for patients at the Brookhaven Laboratories, made the great leap. Cotzias had made leaps before. As a student, he emigrated from Greece to the United States during World War II, and gained acceptance to Harvard Medical School while teaching himself to speak English fluently. Cotzias reasoned that Parkinson's disease should be treatable by increasing the levels of dopamine in the basal ganglia. However, this could not be achieved by directly administering dopamine since this polar molecule does not gain entry into the brain. The so-called blood-brain barrier prevents charged molecules, such as dopamine, from entering the brain itself. Consequently, treatment with dopamine was out of the question. Treatment with tyrosine, a normal dietary constituent that is the precursor for the entire catecholamine pathway (figure 2.3), was unsatisfactory for other reasons. As we have already seen, TH is rate limiting in catecholamine biosynthesis. Consequently, increasing tyrosine will not increase dopamine due to the TH biologic bottleneck. The therapeutic dilemma was clear. How was one to proceed?

Cotzias correctly saw that the solution was L-DOPA therapy (Cotzias et al. 1967). L-DOPA crosses the blood-brain barrier, since it is a nonpolar molecule, and gains access to the dopamine-depleted basal ganglia (caudate). Further, L-DOPA, as the product of the TH enzymatic reaction (figure 2.3), bypasses the rate-limiting step. It may therefore be expected to increase dopamine and improve Parkinsonian signs and symptoms.

Cotzias began his studies with low doses of L-DOPA. Although a number of patients experienced nausea and vomiting, none was relieved of signs and symptoms. Cotzias, however, was tenacious; the principles were sound, and therefore he believed the treatment must ultimately work. He then administered extremely high doses of L-DOPA, and a new era opened in neurology. Patients who had been bedridden or wheelchair bound for years were able to walk. No longer were people foredoomed to an invalid's existence.

The age of molecular therapy in neurology had begun and with it one of the first associations of the molecular and behavioral domains. To begin comprehending the nature of the molecular-behavioral interface, we must take a closer look at the neural systems involved. The action of dopamine in the nigrostriatal system can be undertood schematically by referring to figure 4.4. The globus pallidus, left to its own devices, fosters hyperkinesis, with associated hyperactive movement disorders such as chorea and athetosis. In most of us, the caudate inhibits or suppresses pallidal function, preventing the emergence of

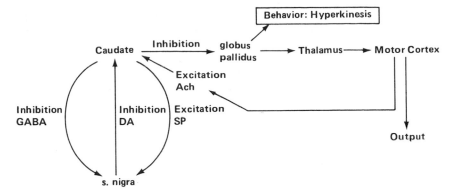

Figure 4.4
The nigrostriatal system: Transmitter organization regulates behavior. Simplified schematic representation of the transmitter organization of the nigrostriatal motor system. Note that under normal circumstances, the caudate inhibits hyperkinetic movement elicited by globus pallidus activation. In this context, the nigrostriatal dopaminergic inhibitory pathway tends to elicit increased movement. Conversely, the cholinergic interneurons of the striatum have a net hypokinetic effect.

GABA = gamma-aminobutyric acid; DA = dopamine; SP = substance P; S. nigra = substantia nigra.

hyperkinesis. In turn, the nigrostriatal pathway, through the mediation of dopamine, inhibits the caudate. The net effect of caudate inhibition, with consequent release of the globus pallidus, is to increase movement. These complex inhibitory and excitatory relationships, mediated by molecules such as dopamine, typify mechanisms at the molecular-behavioral interface.

We are now in a position to understand Parkinson's disease, the central role of dopamine, and, more generally, molecular function and behavior of the organism. In this disease the nigrostriatal system degenerates, decreasing dopaminergic innervation of the caudate and thereby increasing caudate inhibition of globus pallidus. The net effect of dopamine depletion is slowed movements, muscle rigidity, a masklike face, abnormal gait, and all the other associated abnormalities of Parkinson's disease. L-DOPA treatment reverses many of the most debilitating abnormalities by increasing dopamine in the remaining nigrostriatal neurons.

In summary, Cotzias correctly saw that in the nigrostriatal system, dopamine functions as a hyperkinetic agent, relieving the Parkinsonian patient. Cotzias's vision of a molecular therapy for a motor behavioral disorder was vindicated dramatically. Put simply, a single transmitter is capable of altering an abnormal behavioral repertoire.

TH, our prototypical symbolic molecule, occupies a pivotal position in dopamine biosynthesis, directly homologous to that in NE biosynthesis. TH, the rate-limiting enzyme, governs dopamine biosynthesis and thereby is a key determinant of the amount of amine available to function in the caudate (see McGeer et al. 1973; Lerner et al. 1977; Gioguieff 1976, as examples). The critical role of TH has been dramatically demonstrated in the clinical setting. As would be predicted, inhibitors of the enzyme, such as α-methylparatyrosine, cause the emergence of a Parkinsonian-like syndrome. Of greater import therapeutically, however, is the fact that TH inhibitors can alleviate the symptoms of increased movement (hyperkinesis) that occur in chorea or athetosis. These observations follow directly from our previous considerations (for general discussion, see Fahn 1982).

In another parallel, stimuli that increase impulse flow in the nigrostriatal system also cause TH induction with elevated dopamine synthesis (Murrin et al. 1976; Goldstein et al. 1976). Although the physiologic consequences of TH induction in this system have yet to be explored fully, one would predict the emergence of hyperkinetic syndromes. Further, considerations of proximodistal axonal transport of TH from nigra to striatum lead to the prediction of delayed and prolonged effects, as in the locus coeruleus. These contentions have not yet been fully tested experimentally.

Form and Content in Behavior

We have now examined TH in multiple neural systems, peripherally and centrally, to define molecule-systems-behavior relations. A number of generalizations have emerged—some anticipated, others surprising. In the molecular domain of enzyme disinhibition, activation, and induction, remarkable similarity exists in TH among different functional neural systems. For example, increased impulse activity induces TH in all systems examined, regardless of physiologic function. Such striking similarity in a multistep process involving membrane ion flux, elevated TH mRNA, and presumed increased protein synthesis suggests that there are fundamental organizational similarities of molecular function in these different neural systems. A priori there would be little reason to assume an apparent identity of process in cells that differ embryologically, anatomically, and functionally. We shall certainly want to determine whether other mind-brain symbolic molecules, present in diverse neural systems, also exhibit apparent uniformity of regulatory mechanisms.

Although it is unclear how the similarities of mechanism evolved, the consequences of the similarities are unmistakable. Although the different catecholaminergic systems, including sympathoadrenal axis, locus coeruleus, and nigrostriatum, subserve entirely different behavioral functions, similarities of form may be evident. That is, entirely different behavioral contents may exhibit common characteristics of form, including time of onset, duration, and decay, dictated by common regulatory mechanisms governing TH and related catecholaminergic molecular processes. Thus, TH as a prototype is not only necessary for the expression of appropriate behavioral content of a neural system but also shapes the behavior itself. In summary, systems subserving wholly different behaviors may exhibit common characteristics due to use of common molecular symbols.

More generally elucidation of molecular mechanisms underlying the function of neural subsystems may allow the formal classification of behaviors and mental states into form and content. At the very least we may be able to resolve cognitive function into component variables, such as temporal parameters and the behavioral repertoire itself. Such an approach helps place analysis of behavior, both experimental and naturalistic, on a precise, quantitative footing; we may draw closer to solving an unrecognized categorical problem lurking in our midst.

No problem is more illustrative than that of memory. Is memory a discrete cognitive function with a specific neuroanatomic localization or a process exhibited by many neural systems, based on underlying molecular mechanisms? In the latter case, do many different neural systems, serving diverse behavioral functions, undergo changes in state that persist in time, long outlasting the inciting stimulus?

Reexamination of the locus coeruleus from the perspective of mnemonic function may be particularly instructive. For all the roles attributed to it over the years, no one, to my knowledge, has christened the locus as the neural system of memory. I have summarized data supporting the contention that the locus is involved in an arousal-vigilance complex, the postulated "content" of locus function. Closer inspection, however, reveals a clear mnemonic character in locus action. Focusing again on TH induction as a critical hallmark, we can characterize a process of rapid onset, high specificity, and prolonged duration in which repetitive stimuli evoke a progressively greater response, and in which decay occurs in days to weeks. Indeed, in locus terminals in the frontal cortex, TH induction reaches a maximum at approximately two weeks, and activity has returned to basal levels by three and a half weeks (figure 4.2). The same considerations apply to the peripheral sympathetic system, which participates in the fight-or-flight reaction but also exhibits mnemonic traits.

To summarize, by analyzing molecular and behavioral functions simultaneously, we can resolve behavioral and mental states into form and content. Memory factors out as a behavioral form, determined in this instance by the function of specific symbolic molecules. Behavioral content, in contrast, is systems function based on other aspects of organization of the nervous system.

Our discussion illustrates that even based on the unidimensional consideration of a single molecule, TH, we can take the first tentative steps toward the resolution of behavior and mental states into characteristic categories. Subsequent examination of additional symbols will buttress and extend our formulation. A brief consideration of the implications at this juncture may not be premature. Our formulation may help direct theoretical constructs and experimental strategies. Based on experimentation with several different central and peripheral neural systems, we can divide behaviors (and mental states) into content and form. The content of a system's behavior is dictated by neuroanatomic and neurophysiologic organization and consists of such complexes as flight or fight, arousal, and motor coordination. In contrast, each of the underlying neural systems is endowed with memory functions and may be capable of learning, forgetting, and otherwise altering the form of its basic behavioral, physiologic content. A number of implications follow naturally:

> 1. Experimental study of form, such as learning and memory, may be performed with diverse systems that subserve entirely different physiologic functions. We can predict that there are virtually as many memories as physiological molecules and that "new types" of memories will continue to be recognized. The proliferation of "memories" may reflect no more than the recognition of different behavioral contents subject to associated forms.
> 2. Commonalities in forms derived from different subsystems may have more to do with the molecules and subcellular processes involved than with the behavior itself. The taxonomy of behavioral contents may be entirely different from the taxonomy of forms.
> 3. Conversely, apparent similarities in behavioral contents of different subsystems imply little, a priori, about the symbols involved. While common symbols potentially confer similar forms, they do not intrinsically confer similarities of content.
> 4. Search for the exclusive memory mechanism, as an example, may be ill conceived. Different processes characterized by rapid onset, specificity, relatively long-term storage, retrieval, and decay may occur through entirely different molecular mechanisms in different neural systems. Classification will depend on identification of common mechanism, time constants, and so forth.

5. Although form and content can be distinguished in principle, the same molecules participate in both functions. Consequently, for example, inhibition of TH will derange the form and the content of sympathetic, coeruleal, or nigrostriatal function. In at least some systems, then, it may be difficult to resolve form and content with particular experimental strategies.

Chapter 5

Combinatorial Strategies at the Synapse

Combinatorics and Multiple Co-localized Transmitters— Electrochemical Coding—Dopamine/Cholecystokinin, Nucleus Accumbens, and Schizophrenia—Environmental Regulation of Differential Transmitter Expression—Organization of Chemical Circuits

By focusing on specific transducer molecules, we have explored some of the bases for the remarkable specificity, precision, and flexibility exhibited by the nervous system. Yet we have only begun to approach some of the central questions concerning function of the nervous system. How does a rigidly wired, genetically determined nervous system possess the flexibility to receive, encode, store, and retrieve a virtually endless and varying stream of environmental information? Stated differently, what mechanisms allow epigenetic stimuli to alter the structure and function of the brain? How is sufficient diversity generated by a system composed of a finite, and rather limited, number of circuits?

Several recent discoveries are relevant to these questions. Neurons appear to use multiple, co-localized transmitter signals, providing extraordinary potential for combinations of signals even in the single neuron and at the single synapse (for comprehensive review, see Hokfelt et al. 1986). Environmental stimuli appear to regulate the amount and release of different co-localized transmitters independently, allowing experience to become encoded in unique combinations of molecular messages and signals. Additionally different patterns of electrical transmission differentially release different co-localized transmitters and transmitter combinations, constituting a new mechanism, electrochemical coding (Bartfai et al. 1986). The information contained in different impulse patterns is also stored differently in different transmitters, providing a rich molecular source for memory mechanisms.

These few examples define mechanisms that free the nervous system from rigid, genetic, hard-wiring constraints, allowing experience to play a critical role in molecular, cellular, and network systems function. Similar anatomic circuits support different chemical communication pathways at different times, depending on environmental experience. Consequently this new view emphasizes that new chemical networks may be formed in the absence of "structural" neurite elongation, pathfinding, and neosynaptogenesis.

These recently recognized mechanisms, then, constitute a combinatorial strategy in which a limited number of co-localized transmitters are used in varying combinations by neurons to generate diversity. Since transmitter regulation depends on environmental stimuli, molecular mechanisms are able to translate external events and conditions directly into neural information. Remarkably, this processing occurs at the level of the individual neuron, and even the individual synapse.

Use of multiple transmitters in conjunction with plasticity of individual transmitters allows a unique transmitter state to be associated with a specific, complex environmental stimulus. Innervation of a single neuron by multiple afferents, estimated at 30,000 per cortical pyramidal cell (Bullock 1977), leads to rich combinatorial potentials. Rather simple cell assemblies, with unique individual transmitter patterns, consequently may represent complex stimuli and unique patterns and associations of stimuli, giving rise to a rich and subtle representational system.

Before discussing underlying molecular mechanisms, it is useful to indicate some of the more prominent potential properties of the combinatorial nervous system and neuron. First, the total transmitter state of a cell, or, more likely, an ensemble of cells, may represent a unique environmental stimulus or experience.

Second, with multiple chemical circuits existing within a single anatomical pathway, representation of a total stimulus complex by only a subset of fragments may occur, with associational recognition transpiring with a minimal number of neuronal units. A single anatomic network may hold manifold chemical pathways and associations, thereby containing vast amounts of patterned information.

Conversely, malfunction or destruction of a single neuron or small groups of neurons will not destroy a complex, multitransmitter representation or state in an array of neurons. The system, with its diversity, is remarkable fault tolerant.

How, in fact, is combinatorial potential expressed in any given set of neurons? What specific transmitter species are involved? What environmental events govern combinatorial operations? What fundamental processes in the neuron underlying the plasticity are necessary for combinatorial processing?

The background for consideration of combinatorial mechanisms derives from recent work. Contrary to classical teaching, overwhelming evidence now indicates that co-localization of multiple transmitters to individual neurons is widespread, if not universal (table 5.1; Hokfelt et al. 1986). Co-localization occurs in every neuron type regardless of morphology, embryonic origin, or neuropsychologic function (table 5.1). Moreover, co-localized transmitters represent a wide spectrum of chemical classes, including catecholamines, acetylcholine, peptides, purines, and amino acids (table 5.1). How do environmental factors regulate the release of different transmitter combinations, thereby translating diverse environmental conditions and stimuli into differential neuronal signaling?

Electrochemical Coding

It has long been recognized that impulse frequency regulates the amount of transmitter released at well-characterized synapses. For example, at the neuromuscular junction, increased frequency leads to a rise in the quanta of acetylcholine released with increased muscle stimulation and muscle contraction (Katz 1969). In this instance, however, the chemical species released presumably changes only quantitatively, not qualitatively. The realization that multiple transmitters are released by individual neurons raised the possibility that different transmitters, and different combinations of transmitters, are released at different times and different locations by the same neuron. This possibility has been documented experimentally, illustrating the vast combinatorial potential of the individual synapse and the individual neuron.

Frequency of stimulation regulates the chemical nature of the transmitter released in a wide variety of neural systems, centrally and peripherally. In the majority of classical transmitter-peptide neurons, release of peptide is elicited by higher frequencies of stimulation than that required for the release of the classical transmitter alone or in combination. Generally a frequency greater than 2 Hz is required for neuropeptide release, whereas classical transmitter release is evoked by lower rates of stimulation (figure 5.1; Bartfai et al. 1986).

The relationships depicted in figure 5.1 indicate that at very low rates of stimulation, a neuron may act as a purely classical transmitter-releasing cell, at very high rates as a purely peptidergic cell, and in a varying combinatorial fashion at intermediate frequencies. (All of these frequencies fall within the physiologic range.) Consequently by

Table 5.1
Some examples of coexistence of classical neurotransmitters and peptide transmitters
(after Hokfelt et al. 1986)

Classical transmitter	Peptide	Brain region
Dopamine	CCK	Ventral mesencephalon
	Neurotensin	Ventral mesencephalon
		Hypothalamic arcuate nucleus
Norepinephrine	Enkephalin	Locus coeruleus
	NPY	Medulla oblongata
	Vasopressin	Locus coeruleus
Epinephrine	Neurotensin	Medulla oblongata
	NPY	Medulla oblongata
	Substance P	Medulla oblongata
	Neurotensin	Solitary tract nucleus
	CCK	Solitary tract nucleus
5-HT	Substance P	Medulla oblongata
	TRH	Medulla oblongata
	Substance P+TRH	Medulla oblongata
	CCK	Medulla oblongata
	Enkephalin	Medulla oblongata, pons
		Area postrema
ACh	Enkephalin	Superior olive
		Spinal cord
	Substance P	Pons
	VIP	Cortex
	Galanin	Basal forebrain
	CGRP	Medullary motor nuclei
GABA	Motilin(?)	Cerebellum
	Somatostatin	Thalamus
		Cortex, hippocampus
	CCK	Cortex
	NPY	Cortex
	Galanin	Hypothalamus
	Enkephalin	Retina
		Ventral pallidum
	Opioid peptide	Basal ganglia
Glycine	Neurotensin	Retina

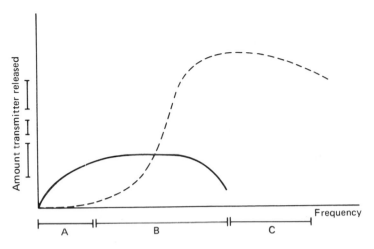

Figure 5.1
Electrochemical coding. Dependence of the chemical nature of the signal on frequency
of stimulation. Schematic illustration of the release of a classical (—) and a peptide (---)
neurotransmitter from a neuron at various frequencies of stimulation. In range A (low
frequency of stimulation), the neuron releases mainly the classical neurotransmitter, in
range B, both neurotransmitters are released, and in range C (high frequency of stimulation) the neuron may act as a peptidergic neuron. (From Bartfai et al. 1986)

altering impulse frequency and pattern, environmental stimuli may
directly alter the nature of the chemical messages released by a neuron
and, as a result, the nature of the information communicated.

Specific examples of electrochemical coding may indicate some of
the mechanisms involved in the newly discovered process. One co-
localized transmitter pair that has received extensive experimental
attention is that of acetylcholine and vasoactive intestinal polypeptide
(VIP). The relationship of these transmitters and the regulation of their
release have been examined in bipolar cells of the cerebral cortex and
in postsynaptic neurons of the cat and rat submandibular salivary
glands (see Bartfai et al. 1986; figure 5.2). Acute excitation (disinhibition) leads to release of acetylcholine. In these systems, acetylcholine
inhibits the release of VIP so that acute stimulation predominantly
releases acetylcholine alone. In contrast, chronic excitation (disinhibition) releases VIP as well as acetylcholine. In these transmitter systems, then, chronic versus acute stimulation qualitatively changes the
nature of the chemical messages that are sent. Moreover, acetylcholine
and VIP exert different physiologic effects that nevertheless are often
complementary.

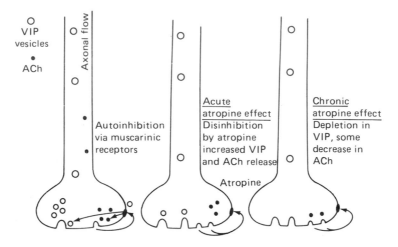

Figure 5.2
An example of the combinatorial neuron: Acetylcholine and VIP. Schematic model for
development of depletion of VIP levels in the submandibularis (and development of
supersensitivity of VIP receptors), in a neuron showing coexistence of ACh and VIP,
upon treatment with the muscarinic antagonist, atropine. Left panel: Control situation,
muscarinic autoinhibition of both ACh and VIP-release is effective. Middle panel: Acute
atropine causes enhanced release. Right panel: Axonal flow cannot keep up with the
increased release; local ACh synthesis partly balances the increased ACh release during
chronic treatment. (From Bartfai et al. 1986)

Additional processes complicate the relationships, leading to even
more complex combinatorial interactions. Long-term chronic stimulation depletes neuronal VIP apparently because ongoing release out-
paces the synthesis of VIP and its transport to nerve terminals. In
contrast, acetylcholine synthesis is able to keep pace with release more
readily. In brief, chronic stimulation results in the release of different
ratios of transmitters depending on duration of the inciting stimuli
(figure 5.2).

Yet another element of complexity is present, since the co-localized
transmitters interact, resulting in additional combinatorial mechanisms. Acetylcholine inhibits the release of VIP by interacting with
specific receptors localized to the neuron itself (autoreceptors) (figure
5.2). Conversely, VIP inhibits the release of acetylcholine by binding
to neuronal VIP receptors. It is apparent that the transmitter, or combinations of transmitters, ultimately released depends on the specific
frequency and pattern of nerve impulses and the character of the
interaction of released transmitters with appropriate autoreceptors.

Since these various processes transpire with different time constants, information may be transmitted and stored over different periods of time under different circumstances.

Electrochemical coding and multiple transmitter interactions appear to be widespread and are certainly not restricted to acetylcholine/VIP-containing neurons. In another example, brainstem raphé neurons contain co-localized serotonin (5-HT) and the peptide, substance P (SP; figure 5.3) In this system 5-HT enhances the depolarization-elicited release of SP from nerve terminals that project to the spinal cord. This effect is blocked by specific 5-HT antagonists, establishing its specificity (Bartfai et al. 1986). Conversely, SP evokes 5-HT release from terminals autoinhibited by 5-HT itself (Mitchell and Fleetwood-Walker 1981), indicating the complexity of intertransmitter relationships, and the potential for rich combinatorial information transfer (figure 5.3).

How do co-localization and electrochemical coding translate into behavior? The peptide cholecystokinin (CCK) and the catecholamine

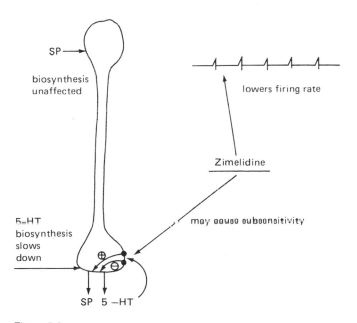

Figure 5.3
A cooperative combinatorial neuron: Serotonin and substance P. In this instance, the drug zimelidine, through action at different sites, may result in increased substance P in terminals in the ventral spinal cord of the descending neurons.
SP = substance P; 5-HT = serotonin.

dopamine (DA) are co-localized to the mesolimbic system in the brain (figure 5.4). The DA/CCK neurons of the ventral mesencephalon project to a number of limbic structures, most importantly the nucleus accumbens, olfactory tubercle, and central nucleus of the amygdala (Hokfelt et al. 1980a, 1980b). This system has been of particular interest since hyperactivity of this dopaminergic pathway has been invoked as a key element in the pathogenesis of schizophrenia (see chapter 10). Extensive electrophysiologic and pharmacologic studies indicate that CCK enhances the actions of DA in this system (Meyer and Krause 1983; Fuxe et al. 1981; Crawley et al. 1985). What are the behavioral sequelae of these specific transmitter interactions? In fact, CCK exerts notable effects on DA-mediated behaviors (for review, see Skirboll et al. 1986). DA released in the rat accumbens is known to elicit hyperlocomotion and stereotypy, two schizophreniform behaviors (figure 5.4). Similarly, administration of CCK along with apomorphine, a potent DA agonist, markedly increases the stereotypy evoked by apomorphine alone (Crawley 1985). These effects are specific for the agents employed and are restricted to the accumbens anatomically. Clearly co-localization and combinatorial processing have profound behavioral as well as biochemical consequences.

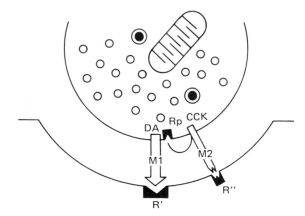

Figure 5.4
Mesolimbic neurons, combinatorial effects, and schizophreniform behavior. Schematic representation of a nerve ending that contains both dopamine (DA) and cholecystokinin (CCK). In this instance, CCK may inhibit the release of DA by action on presynaptic receptors. Both dopamine and CCK have been implicated in schizophreniform behavior. (After Hokfelt et al. 1986)

Combinatorial Transmitter Storage

Having surveyed some of the implications of electrochemical coding, we now briefly examine some of the cellular biological mechanisms underlying combinatorial processing. A more detailed understanding may provide further insights into the nature of the synapse and the nature of communication itself in the nervous system. Transmitters are stored in "packets" or vesicles within nerve terminals, and the vesicles release their contents in response to nerve impulses. In many instances, co-localized transmitters are also co-stored in the same vesicles. For example, in the adrenal chromaffin model cell, opiate peptides and catecholamines are stored in the same vesicles, and the ratio of transmitters released reflects the ratio of storage in the vesicles (Wilson et al. 1982). A similar situation exists in certain neurons. For example ATP, which serves as a transmitter in some systems, is co-stored, and co-released from some sympathetic nerves and from motor terminals at the neuromuscular junction (for review, see Burnstock 1986).

In contrast, an entirely different mode of storage, leading to wholly novel modes of communication, has recently been identified. In some neuronal populations, different neuronal transmitters localized to the same neuron are stored in separate vesicles. For example, vasopressin and oxytocin are stored in different vesicles in hypothalamic magno-cellular neurons (Brownstein and Mezey 1986). Similarly, the transmitter pair acetylcholine and VIP, or norepinephrine and neuropeptide Y, are co-localized to the same autonomic neurons but stored in different vesicles (Hokfelt et al. 1986; Lundberg and Hokfelt 1986; Stjarne and Lundberg 1986). Further, some populations of vesicles in the same neurons do co-store the transmitters (Stjarne and Lundberg 1986). It is apparent that populations of neurons have the built-in capacity to translate patterns of impulse activity into patterns of release with exquisite precision. Many neurons and synapses appear to be designed to maximize flexibility of communication through combinatorial mechanisms. Concepts of the rigid, digital synapse are clearly inadequate and even misleading in the analysis of neural information transfer. Differential storage provides at least one mechanism for qualitative as well as quantitative changes in transmitters released in response to different environmental stimuli.

Closely related to the process of differential storage and release are the processes of differential expression and metabolism of co-localized transmitters. These processes add a further dimension to electrochemical coding and combinatorial processing and extend our concepts of information transfer at the synapse.

Differential Transmitter Expression and Metabolism

Environmental stimuli not only regulate the chemical nature of the transmitters released but also govern the transmitter phenotype of a neuron. Different environmental signals elicit the de novo expression of new transmitters in neurons. More precisely, the environment appears to regulate phenotypic expression at the most fundamental level in the neuron: gene readout. Through this mechanism, neurons exhibit the capability to store environmental information for relatively long periods of time, bridging the temporal gap between the short-term effects of electrochemical coding in the regulation of release and longer-term changes in the actual expression of transmitter phenotypes.

A variety of signals influence transmitter phenotypic expression. For example, experiments performed in vivo indicate that microenvironmental characters of different brain regions alter neuronal phenotype. In one series of experiments, transplantation of neurons to the mammalian brain differentially influences transmitter expression (Schultzberg et al. 1986). Mesencephalic raphé 5-HT neurons express SP de novo when transplanted to the hippocampus or striatum, but not after transplantation to the spinal cord. Presumably region-specific microenvironmental factors in the brain regulate the transmitter mix expressed by defined neurons.

Long-range humoral factors also regulate the messages elaborated by certain neurons. The parvocellular neurons of the hypothalamus are responsive to adrenal glucocorticoid hormones. In this neuronal population, glucocorticoids decrease the production of corticotrophin releasing factor (CRF), vasopressin, and angiotensin II through a negative feedback mechanism, but do not alter the production of enkephalin or neurotensin (Swanson et al. 1986).

It is apparent that a variety of epigenetic, extracellular signals regulate transmitter expression, thereby providing mechanisms for the relatively long-term storage of information. What neuronal molecular mechanisms actually underlie plasticity of expression? A number of these processes are being defined in the relatively simple sympathetic neuron, which we have already discussed. Moreover, similar regulatory events appear to transpire in brain neurons as well, indicating that common molecular mechanisms are utilized by central as well as peripheral neurons.

I have already discussed the catecholaminergic transmitter system in detail and need only summarize several salient points. TH, the rate-limiting enzyme in catecholamine biosynthesis, is a critical index of catecholamine expression and metabolism. Transsynaptic stimulation of sympathetic neurons results in the induction of TH, an increase in the number of molecules, leading to an increase in enzyme catalytic activity and in catecholamine biosynthesis.

What molecular mechanisms transduce impulse activity into TH induction? An increase in molecule number may, theoretically, result from increased enzyme synthesis or decreased degradation (figures 2.3 and 2.5). Previous work had indicated that inhibitors of protein or RNA synthesis prevented induction of TH, suggesting that increased synthesis mediates the rise of TH. This contention remained circumstantial, however, since the metabolic inhibitors exert multiple direct and indirect effects. The recent availability of a complementary DNA coding for TH allowed direct study of gene expression. In turn, quantitation of message after increased transsynaptic activity might indicate whether synthesis of TH protein by its mRNA is actually elevated by increased impulse activity.

Superior cervical sympathetic ganglion neurons in rats were used as a model system (Black et al. 1985). Increased impulse activity induced TH, as expected, and significantly elevated TH mRNA. Further, denervation of the ganglion prevented the rise in TH and its mRNA, indicating that increased transsynaptic impulse activity per se increased the message (figure 5.5). These results provide more direct evidence that increased impulse frequency increases TH by increasing its synthesis from mRNA.

We can now ask the fundamental question of whether impulse activity, communication in the nervous system, actually regulates the readout of mRNA from genomic DNA. Does the environment govern which genes are expressed, a potentially powerful mechanism for information processing in the nervous system? In the sympathetic system, the definitive answer is not available. Although pharmacologic inhibitors of gene readout prevent TH induction by increased impulse activity, suggesting that the regulation of gene transcription is involved, this approach is indirect; measures of transcription itself are required. Nevertheless, evidence is certainly consistent with the regulation of gene readout by depolarization, which has recently been demonstrated in another model system, the adrenal medulla.

In summary, impulse activity regulates the expression of specific, critical transmitter molecules, and this effect is mediated by the alteration of levels of specific encoding message, probably through selective changes in gene readout. In terms of combinatorial potential, we should want to know whether TH molecule number is a continuous function of impulse activity such that different frequencies elicit different concentrations of molecules, leading to a continuum of molecule

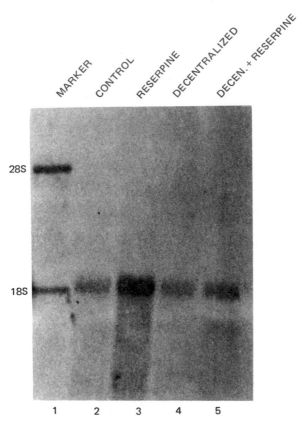

Figure 5.5
Impulse activity regulates levels of transmitter (TH) mRNA. Northern blot analysis of
TH mRNA in superior cervical ganglia. Marker lane, 18S and 28S ribosomal RNA;
control, vehicle treated and intact; reserpine, reserpine treatment and intact; decen-
tralized, denervated and vehicle treated; decen. plus reserpine, denervated and reserpine treated. (From Black et al. 1985)

numbers. In brief, do multiple states occur, or is this an all-or-none phenomenon?

In fact, recent discoveries indicate that TH molecule numbers vary over a virtually continuous range, depending on impulse frequency and stimulus repetition. In one group of studies, rats were treated with the pharmacologic agent reserpine, which mimics environmental stress by increasing sympathetic impulse activity (Mueller et al. 1969). A single dose evoked a 2.5-fold increase in TH in three days. In contrast, repeated daily treatment for five days elicited a 5-fold rise. Direct electrical stimulation of the innervating nerves paralleled these results. Stimulation at 20 Hz for only 10 minutes increased TH activity 25 percent three days later, and stimulation for 60 minutes increased enzyme activity by 73 percent (Zigmond and Chalazonitis 1979; Zigmond et al. 1980) Consequently, repetition and increased stimulus duration cause a progressive increase in TH, maximizing combinatorial potential. Note that these stimulus-response characteristics define the rudiments of a memory mechanism (Black et al. 1987).

How do other transmitters, localized to the same sympathetic neurons, respond to transsynaptic stimulation? What is the effect on the combinatorial potential of this simple, well-defined system? The putative peptide transmitter, substance P (SP), has recently been localized to sympathetic neurons and exerts electrophysiological effects entirely different from those of norepinephrine. SP iontophoresis elicits a slow excitatory postsynaptic potential (Dun and Karczmar 1979), whereas norepinephrine is either inhibitory or modulatory (for review, see Cooper et al. 1982). Consequently any differential in transsynaptic regulation of TH and SP would result in a marked combinatorial potential of the sympathetic neuron, with marked variation in target responses.

In fact, extensive experiments indicate that impulse activity suppresses SP in sympathetic neurons, thereby exerting an effect opposite to that on TH (figure 5.6). For example, denervation of sympathetic ganglia in adult rats or pharmacologic blockade of ganglionic transmission elevates SP in sympathetic neurons (Kessler et al. 1981; Kessler and Black 1982). Conversely increased impulse activity, elicited pharmacologically, decreases SP. These observations in live animals suggest that impulse activity decreases SP, an effect diametrically opposed to that on TH (figure 5.6).

Increased impulse activity tends to increase norepinephrine, an inhibitory transmitter, while decreasing excitatory SP. Restated, different impulse frequencies result in different transmitter ratios in sympathetic neurons, with different target effects. What molecular mechanisms underlie this differential regulation that leads to combi-

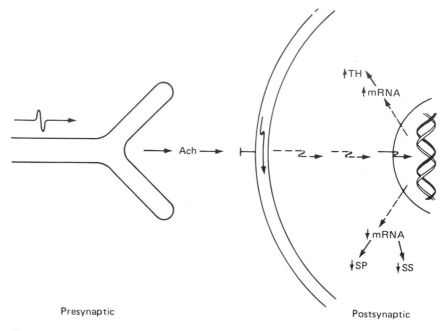

Presynaptic   Postsynaptic

Figure 5.6
Environment differentially regulates co-localized transmitters. Transsynaptic impulse
activity increases catecholaminergic function by increasing mRNA coding for tyrosine
hydroxylase. Simultaneously, increased impulse activity decreases co-localized peptidergic function by reducing messengers coding for the putative transmitters, substance
P and somatostatin.

natorial processing within the single neuron? Is the potential for combinatorial processing of neural signals intrinsic to the individual
neuron, or is it a result of higher-order interactions?

Counterintuitively, perhaps, the machinery for the transduction of
environmental signals into combinatorial information is built into the
individual neuron and involves a most fundamental level, the neuronal genome. These insights have largely been derived from analysis
of combinatorial processing in simplified, rigorously controlled tissue
culture systems. Explantation of ganglia to culture, with consequent
denervation, results in a ten-fold rise in SP within a day, and a forty-
fold increase in four to six days that is maintained for at least a month
(Kessler et al. 1981, 1983). Moreover, depolarization in culture reproduces the effect of impulse activity in vivo, preventing the increase in
SP. Further, tetrodotoxin, which blocks depolarization by preventing

Na^+ influx, apparently simultaneously increases TH and depresses SP (figure 5.6).

The mirror-image, regulatory symmetry extends to the molecular genetic mechanisms underlying the reciprocal regulation of SP and TH. I have already indicated that the transsynaptic induction of TH is associated with elevation of specific TH mRNA, which may be due to enhanced gene readout. Ongoing work now indicates that the increase in SP peptide is also associated with increased preprotachykinin mRNA, message coding for the SP precursor protein (Roach et al. 1987). Consequently, to a first approximation, levels of regulation of TH and SP appear to be similar, the elaboration of specific mRNA (figure 5.6). The effects of depolarization on preprotachykinin gene transcription are being examined to determine whether impulse activity regulates peptide gene readout itself.

In summary, synaptic impulse activity is represented by mirror-image changes in the numbers of specific molecules associated with two different transmitters. The relatively simple sympathetic neuron exhibits a wide variety of combinatorial states in response to impulse activity. Do any other transmitters in sympathetic neurons exhibit changes with depolarizing stimuli?

Although evidence is still fragmentary, another peptide, somato-statin (SS), has been identified in the same sympathetic neurons and varies with depolarizing influences (Kessler et al. 1983). Explantation of ganglia results in a marked rise in SS, paralleling the increase in SP. Moreover, depolarizing influences block the increase in SS in a tetro-dotoxin-preventable manner, further mimicking SP regulation. On-going studies are now characterizing underlying mechanisms in detail to provide a more fully integrated picture of combinatorial processing in this model neuron. These initial observations, however, suggest that at least three different transmitters may code in a combinatorial fashion for impulse activity.

While regulation of the foregoing transmitters comprises a rich com-binatorial system, emerging evidence indicates that multiple addi-tional transmitters are also localized to sympathetic neurons, leading to a vast combinatorial potential. For example, sympathetic neurons also express leucine- and methionine-enkephalin, adenosine, neuro-peptide Y, cholecystokinin, lutenizing hormone releasing hormone (LHRH), VIP, and a vasopressin-like molecule (for review, see Hanley 1989a, 1989b). The role of these transmitters in the representational, combinatorial process remains to be defined.

Transmitters in the sympathetic system are semantically as well as syntactically functional. That is, transmitter symbols exert well-doc-umented physiologic effects in a neural system that governs vegetative functions. Consequently any given transmitter state translates into specific cardiovascular, respiratory, gastrointestinal, and genitourinary functions, for example. Thus, the same molecules that regulate physiologic function simultaneously transduce, integrate, store, and express information concerning impulse activity. This multifunctional use of transducer molecules obviates the need to posit the existence of separate and distinct information-bearing (cognitive) structures. We shall certainly want to know whether this principle is operative in higher brain centers.

Even in the sympathetic system, investigations have just begun. We now must precisely define relations underlying chemical coding. How exactly are transmitter states related to impulse frequency and temporospatial patterning of impulses? How do specific environmental stimuli regulate impulse activity in this system that is concerned with responses to stress and to emergency? Answers to these questions may allow us to relate specific external stimuli to impulse pattern and to the specific encoding transmitter state.

Regardless of precise answers to these questions, it is apparent that functions that might be termed cognitive, such as persistence of altered state with time, increased symbol magnitude with repetitive stimuli, and representation of a stimulus by a neuronal symbol itself, all occur in the peripheral sympathetic neuron. Consequently the fundamental units used for such cognitive functions as memory are apparent in this peripheral system. In this sense, it is clear that critical units of cognitive functions are present in diverse subsystems and are not restricted to particular cerebral centers. We may anticipate that different telencephalic areas use these basic molecular mechanisms in the elaboration of increasingly complex cognitive phenomena.

Combinatorial Systems in the Adrenal Medulla Model System

In initial attempts to ascertain the prevalence of combinatorial, representational processes, we continue examination of accessible peripheral systems by focusing on the adrenal medulla. This model system broadens our inquiry in several critical aspects. First, these cells, closely related to neurons, function in the endocrine mode, releasing molecular signals into the circulation. Second, the actual signals employed are different, in part, from those elaborated by sympathetics, allowing us to determine whether different signals, derived from different precursor molecules, and encoded in different genes, follow similar combinatorial principles. By extending our view to the endocrine system and hormonal signals, we can determine whether the combinatorial representational strategy underlies distant as well as proximate intercellular signaling and whether, consequently, the strategy extends beyond the nervous system. Ubiquity, in turn, may provide clues concerning phylogeny of the process. The adrenal medulla is a particularly apt model in the context of this discussion since chromaffin cells receive a cholinergic innervation, paralleling principal sympathetic neurons. Does impulse activity govern humoral patterns in the adrenal medulla, as in sympathetics?

The medullary chromaffin cells have long been known to elaborate and secrete the catecholamines, norepinephrine and epinephrine (for review, see Iversen 1967, p. 30). Recent studies indicate that leucine- and methionine-enkephalin are co-stored and co-released with the catecholamines (Viveros et al. 1979; Livett et al. 1981; Govoni et al. 1981). Leu- and met-enkephalin are derived from the same preproenkephalin precursor polypeptide molecule, and radioimmunoassay of either may be used to monitor opiate peptide status. In turn, TH may be used as an index of catecholamine regulation in general, and PNMT, the enzyme that converts norepinephrine to epinephrine, may be used to monitor adrenergic status specifically.

In fact, combinatorial patterns and underlying mechanisms are strikingly similar in medulla and sympathetic neurons. Denervation of the adrenal medulla in adults markedly increases leu-enk (Bohn et al. 1983; LaGamma et al. 1985). Further, blockade of cholinergic transmission pharmacologically reproduces the effect of surgical denervation, indicating that cholinergic-induced depolarization itself regulates leu-enk (these results are strikingly similar to those described for SP in sympathetic neurons). Neither surgical denervation nor pharmacologic blockade affected activities of TH or PNMT. Nevertheless, it has long been known that both enzymes are subject to transsynaptic induction by increased impulse activity. Consequently, as in sympathetics, the catecholamine and peptide transmitters appear to be differentially regulated.

Governing molecular and molecular genetic mechanisms have been examined in greater detail by explanting the adult medulla to culture, following the strategy employed with sympathetic neurons. In summary, explantation, with consequent denervation, results in a fifty-fold rise in leu-enk within four days (LaGamma et al. 1984). TH is unchanged, and PNMT decreases 60 percent to new, stable plateau values. Further, depolarization with veratridine completely prevents the dramatic increase in leu-enk in a tetrodotoxin-preventable manner, further mimicking results in sympathetics. In essence, then, transsynaptic impulses and medullary depolarization (and/or its sequelae) suppress leu-enk; these processes are known to induce medullary TH and PNMT. Consequently, similar combinatorial patterns are generated in adrenal and sympathetics by impulse activity. Can we begin to delineate underlying molecular genetic mechanisms?

In pilot studies in culture, inhibition of protein synthesis with cycloheximide completely blocks the increase in leu-enk, while inhibition of RNA synthesis with actinomycin D or α-amanitin inhibits the rise by 50 percent (LaGamma et al. 1985). Consequently both ongoing protein and RNA synthesis are necessary for the normal increase in leu-enk. The availability of a preproenkephalin cDNA probe allows definition of the level of regulation directly.

To determine whether the increase in leu-enk was associated with a rise in mRNA coding for the opiate peptide precursor molecule, preproenkephalin mRNA levels were determined after four days in culture. There was a striking increase in preproenkephalin mRNA compared to freshly dissected (zero time) medullae (LaGamma et al. 1985).

To characterize the apparent increase in preproenkephalin mRNA in greater detail, more detailed analysis was performed. After explantation, preproenkephalin mRNA increased progressively: analysis revealed a 34-fold rise after two days and a 74-fold increase after four days of culture.

To determine whether depolarization itself altered levels of preproenkephalin mRNA, medullae were cultured in the presence of depolarizing agents. Exposure to elevated potassium inhibited the increase in mRNA at two days. Moreover, the depolarizing agent veratridine, which increases transmembrane sodium ion flux, reproduced the effects of potassium, inhibiting the rise in preproenkephalin mRNA. Tetrodotoxin, which antagonized the effects of veratridine on sodium ion channels, prevented the effects of veratridine on preproenkephalin mRNA.

In aggregate, these observations strongly suggest that depolarization regulates medullary leu-enk by altering levels of preproenkephalin mRNA. Parallel experiments indicate that preproenkephalin mRNA increases 34-fold after two days in culture, prior to any detectable increase in leu-enk. At four days when leu-enk has increased markedly, preproenkephalin mRNA exhibits a 74-fold rise. Viewed in conjunction with the metabolic inhibitor data, it appears that accretion of opiate peptide is mediated, at least in part, by transcription and ongoing translation.

The adrenal medulla model system provided enough tissue to analyze the level of regulation precisely. In fact, by examining gene readout directly (with so-called run-on assays), it is clear the depolarization actually regulates gene transcription. Explantation and denervation elicit a marked increase in preproenkephalin gene expression, and depolarization inhibits gene readout. It is apparent that this is a powerful mechanism for the long-term storage of information in the neuroendocrine cell. A number of critical questions can now be approached. What mechanisms mediate the translation of membrane depolarization into altered gene readout? What is the duration of altered readout with respect to the inciting depolarizing stimuli? Are whole gene families subject to this regulation, and, if so, will this provide hints regarding the overall orchestration of information in the nervous and endocrine systems?

Thus, peripheral neuroendocrine cells utilize molecular signals as symbols to represent impulse activity. Different combinatorial states transduce different impulse frequencies, evoking different physiologic effects. Hormone and transmitter serve the dual roles of physiologic effector and information encoder. Do virtually all cells use and store extracellular (environmental) information in this manner? What are the implications for phylogenetic origins of these processes? Before approaching these issues, we might reexamine the potential for combinatorial representation in the brain.

Combinatorial Potential in the Brain: Mechanistic Considerations

While the relatively simple, accessible periphery has yielded initial insights concerning molecular mechanisms governing combinatorial representation, increasing evidence suggests that similar processes govern neuronal function in the brain. Once again, the nucleus locus coeruleus may serve as an informative model system.

Do locus neurons fulfill the two central criteria: are multiple transmitters elaborated and used, and do transmitters or their regulators change with impulse activity? In fact, locus neurons contain the catecholamine norepinephrine, and subpopulations contain the putative peptide transmitters, neuropeptide Y (NPY) and galanin (Melander et al. 1986; for review, see Gray and Morley 1986). The discoveries of NPY and galanin are so recent that their regulation has yet to be defined. However, studies of the locus catecholaminergic system indicate that TH does indeed change under conditions of stress. More recent studies, performed in cultured locus, indicate that depolarizing stimuli do indeed induce TH; combinatorial potential is present in brain, as well as periphery. A brief description will illustrate the nature of the observations and the gaps in our knowledge.

Cold stress, immobilization stress, and a variety of pharmacologic agents induce TH in the rat locus in vivo, leading to the speculation that depolarization might mediate this effect. Experiments performed with the explanted locus grown in culture are now supporting this contention. Briefly, exposure of the cultured locus to veratridine or depolarizing concentrations of potassium ion increases TH catalytic activity. Moreover, the increase in activity is associated with an increase in TH molecule number (Dreyfus et al. 1986). Consequently the CA system in this brain nucleus may exist in multiple states, governed by depolarization state. Finally, the increase in locus TH is, in fact, accompanied by a rise in mRNA coding for the enzyme (Biguet et al. 1986). In summary, regulation of gene readout in locus by impulse activity may parallel that discovered in peripheral systems. It is now critical to determine whether NPY and galanin are similarly responsive and whether, therefore, multiple transmitter combinatorial states are exhibited.

Interpretations and Implications

Combinatorial strategies within neurons lead to a number of potential combinatorial strategies among neurons, providing an unbroken line of logic from molecular, transmitter symbols to neuron sets and assemblies. The chemical communication between afferent transmitter phenotype and postsynaptic transmitter receptor provides a plastic, chemical circuit impressed on a background of the relatively hard-wired anatomical circuitry of the nervous system. The transmitter symbols that encode information within the neuron also serve as signals to activate postsynaptic neurons. The use of multiple transmitters by neurons vastly expands the potential for spatial pattern formation in the already anatomically complex nervous system. Further, phenotypic plasticity adds a degree of temporal flexibility, allowing chemical circuits to form and dissolve and strengthen and weaken with appropriate use and disuse.

Whereas the hard-wiring blueprint of the nervous system derives predominantly from ontogenetic mechanisms common to a species as a whole, critical aspects of the chemical circuitry may be dependent on the individual's experience. Plasticity of multiple, co-localized transmitters may allow a "prewired" anatomical circuit to change its fundamental character. In behavioral-cognitive terms, it is this plasticity that confers individuality, based on unique inner and outer experiences, in the presence of hard-wired commonality. Embedded within the more or less fixed, species-specified circuits lies the potential for chemically coded patterns that may change form and function based on experience.

It may be useful to specifically define the patterns generated by chemical circuitry to appreciate their salient characteristics. Patterns may be simply classified as topographic or combinatorial, two non-mutually exclusive categories. In the simplest case, the coincidence of a presynaptic transmitter and its postsynaptic receptor allows interaction, regardless of the presence of other transmitters and receptors. Simple topographic coding (figure 5.7) in which afferents chemically match spatially parallel efferents preserves topography and represents the chemical analogue of many sensory (e.g., vision, somethesia) and motor systems. However, in any anatomical simple topographic system, chemical diversity allows parallel processing in discrete chemical pathways, vastly increasing the potential for information flow. Indeed, the dorsal root sensory ganglion in mammals consists of subsets of co-mingling neurons containing different peptide transmitters, allowing precisely for this mode of processing. Moreover, as our database expands, we may be able to detect chemical topography in anatomic systems apparently devoid of such arrangements based on classical anatomic analysis.

Topographic iterative chemical coding (figure 5.7) represents a complex, transitional form between simple topographic and combinatorial and, when extended several synapses beyond, detects specific patterns of environmental stimuli. In topographic iterative patterns, an axon containing transmitters A and B projects through linearly extended sets of dendrites (or somata) containing appropriate receptors A' and B'; parallel patterns occur in C and D and C' and D'. Progressive elaboration of this pattern may result in upstream cells that respond only to the entire combination, ABCD. These more central cells thus recognize complex environmental patterns by responding only to simultaneous stimulation by separate iterative arrays A'B' and C'D' (figure 5.7). Selected characteristics of a stimulus complex are thereby extracted. This line of argument, however, is ultimately dependent on true combinatorial processing.

In its most elemental form, true combinatorial interneuronal processing may be either divergent or convergent at the single relay level. Chemically coded convergence allows the second-order neuron (figure 5.7) to respond to primary neurons that are spatially dispersed and potentially excited by entirely different stimulus features. This situation parallels that described in the previous paragraph, allowing higher-order, more "central" neurons to respond to complex stimuli composed of the elements represented by the first-order neuron symbols. Simple divergence (figure 5.7) allows the symbols in a single first-order afferent to participate in multiple higher-order representations. Complex combinatorial chemical circuits combine these features: a single first-order neuron (or synapse) participates in multiple complex second-order representations and simultaneously is but one of multiple elements converging on other second-order cells to form

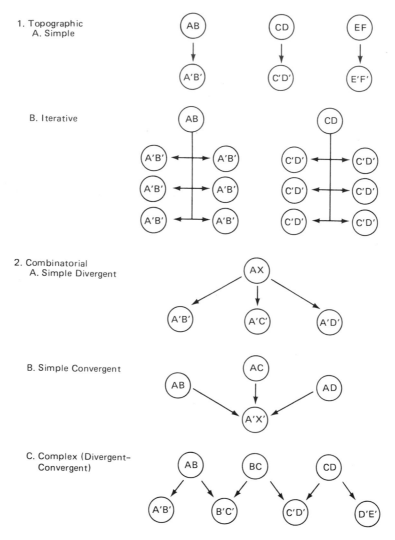

Figure 5.7
Combinatorial coding of circuits. For illustrative purposes circuits may be subdivided into topographic and combinatorial. As an example, simple topographic circuits represent point-to-point communication and may be instantiated in primary sensory and motor systems. In these circuits, presynaptic transmitters correspond to postsynaptic responsivity. Topographic iterative circuits, typified by climbing fibers in the cerebellum, are characterized by afferent fibers that innervate an extended array of receptive neurons. In these systems, all postsynaptic neurons innervated respond to the particular presynaptic transmitters released. In combinatorial systems, a variety of presynaptic-postsynaptic matches occur. In simple divergent systems, one of many presynaptic transmitters may communicate with a variety of postsynaptic neurons through appropriate receptors. Conversely, in simple convergent systems, multiple presynaptic neurons may communicate with a single postsynaptic population due to elaboration of a matching presynaptic transmitter. The complex system combines features of divergent and convergent systems allowing the emergence of unique combinations of circuits.

higher orders of pattern recognition. Further, in the complex pattern (figure 5.7), second-order neurons respond maximally only when both inputs discharge simultaneously, providing the substrate for true associational processing.

Heretofore our formulation has depended on the dual function of transmitters as symbols and signals communicating through conventional (ultramicroscopic) anatomical synapses. However, under certain circumstances, chemical communication may be freed from the constraints imposed by hard-wired circuitry. Different transmitters in the same neuron may elicit responses in different target neurons; some of the target neurons may not even receive anatomical synaptic innervation from the stimulating, afferent neuron. For example, in the bullfrog sympathetic ganglion, presynaptic cholinergic fibers innervate one class of neurons, stimulating them by releasing acetylcholine at the synapse. However, these afferent cholinergic fibers also contain and release an LHRH-like peptide. The peptide diffuses many micrometers before eliciting a slow excitatory postsynaptic potential (EPSP) in an entirely different class of sympathetic neurons, lacking LHRH synapses (for review, see Branton et al. 1986). In this instance, then, neuronal intercommunication occurs through hormonal mechanisms, not true synaptic mediation, dependent on extracellular stability of peptide and peptide receptor on the target cell. Consequently physicochemical properties of the transmitter confer the potential for "unconventional" modes of neural communication. More generally, this is an example of incongruence between anatomic and chemical circuits: specific chemical communication within the nervous system is not restricted to anatomical pathways and anatomical synapses. This frontal attack on neuroanatomic orthodoxy is not without harbinger, if not precedent. It is well recognized that sex steroids and glucocorticoid hormones specifically interact with neuron receptors, evoking physiologic responses. Nevertheless, nonsynaptic communication wholly within the nervous system has not been widely appreciated.

The implications are rather remarkable, if highly speculative. We may view the patterns in figure 5.7 as either structural (anatomic) and/or chemical. In the extreme, cell assemblies, networks, and matrices may be either anatomical or chemical. As a minimum, chemical networks and nonsynaptic communication may complement anatomic circuits and offer rich potential for associative phenomena.

Viewed in the context of transmitter plasticity, nonsynaptic chemical communication allows the formation of new networks and cell assemblies in the absence of neurite elongation, pathfinding, and neosynaptogenesis. Consequently the formation or strengthening of new chemical circuits may not be associated with detectable structural analogues. Conversely similar anatomic patterns may support different chemical communication pathways, presumably elicited by altered external stimuli. At the very least, these arguments caution against drawing conclusions solely on neuroanatomic grounds and prematurely closing accounts with neural network reality.

Chapter 6

Molecules and Modularity of Brain Function

AVP: Antidiuretic, Vasopressor, Transmitter, Hormone—Polyprotein Strategy—POMC: ACTH, Endorphin, MSHs, and Stress Responses— Opioid Peptides—Genomic Organization of Polyproteins—Gene Structure Dictating Modularity—Invertebrate Polyprotein Modules: ELH

Extensive work in neurology, psychology, and neuroscience suggests that brain structure and function are organized into discrete modules (Fodor 1983; Gazzaniga 1989; Pylyshyn 1980). Mental life, an apparently unified experience, actually consists of multiple individual components. Even the seemingly simple psychological act of calling an image to mind involves manifold events in the recall of images from memory and subsequent mental manipulation (Kosslyn 1988). Conclusions based on psychological analysis are complemented by neuroscientific studies. Abundant evidence now indicates that different brain areas subserve different mental functions and that disconnection of areas prevents normal, integrated mind function. Moreover, sensory processing of a stimulus occurs through multiple, parallel pathways. In vision, for example, color, motion, and depth perception are analyzed by different pathways that nevertheless result in apparently unified perception (Livingstone and Hubel 1988). In summary, the concept of modularity is supported by psychological analysis and analysis of functional neuroanatomic organization. **Modularity, however, also derives from a previously unrecognized domain: the genomic and biochemical organization of neuroeffector molecules.**

Neurons synthesize polyfunctional proteins that contain multiple biologically active molecules involved in a module of related behaviors (for example, see figure 6.3). These polyproteins are composed of a sequence of individual peptide molecules, each encoding a different but related behavior. Physiologic digestion of the parent molecule in the cell liberates the components, each of which then elicits its characteristic behavior.

Consequently, these "polyproteins" effectively code for associated behaviors. That is, processing of a single molecule by proteolytic cleavage liberates individual neurohormones that generate the complex, but stereotyped, collection of individual behaviors. Stated another way, a single population of neurons may subserve a number of associated behaviors, each governed by a different transmitter, by synthesizing a single protein. Using this mechanism, then, synthesis of a single protein ensures that a specific, complex behavioral repertoire will occur in an integrated fashion.

We may pose specific questions concerning the polyprotein biological strategy. What polyproteins are known to govern behaviors? How is a single polyprotein converted to the component parts that elicit related behaviors? How do genes code for polyproteins? Does genomic organization provide insight concerning the organization of behavior? Does the polyprotein strategy provide any mechanisms for plasticity? Finally, how widespread is this strategy? Is it restricted to the nervous system; is it widespread phylogenetically?

For illustrative purposes, we begin by examining a single neuroeffector molecule that encodes multiple physiologic actions. Using a relatively simple model molecule, we hope to discern those environmental stimuli that evoke secretion and the battery of actions that are triggered. The relationship of molecule to modularity may be most easily appreciated in a simple system. Subsequently, true polyproteins, which contain different molecules, each governing a discrete physiological-behavioral repertoire, are examined in detail. One of our primary goals is to define the environmental stimuli represented by the molecules and the physiologic behavior into which this information is translated.

Arginine Vasopressin: A Simple Model Molecule

Mammalian arginine vasopressin (AVP) is a simple octapeptide (eight amino acids) that plays a critical role in the regulation of water balance in the body (for review, see Andreoli 1982). The single polypeptide exerts multiple physiologic effects, and its secretion is elicited by specific stimuli (figure 6.1). In brief, AVP secretion is evoked by conditions resulting from reduced total body water, such as decreased intravascular (blood) volume or increased plasma concentration (increased plasma osmotic pressure) and by pain and stress. In turn, AVP exerts a variety of physiological effects, related directly or indirectly to restitution of appropriate fluid balance. Although it is only a single molecule, this polyfunctional protein exerts multiple physiologic effects. The posterior pituitary neurohormone acts directly on

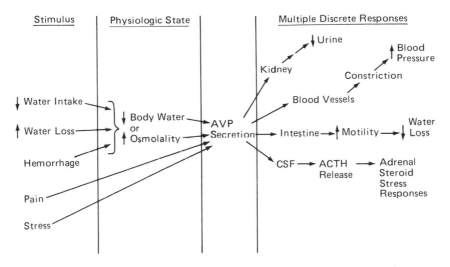

Figure 6.1
A signal polyfunctional protein and information flow: AVP. Schematic representation of the flow of information from environmental or extracellular stimulus to physiologic state to AVP secretion, resulting in discrete physiologic responses.

the kidney as an antidiuretic, decreasing urine formation and water loss. Second, AVP causes blood vessel constriction, thereby maintaining blood pressure in the face of decreased blood volume. Third, the molecule stimulates intestinal motility, presumably altering enteric fluid loss. Finally, AVP released into the cerebrospinal fluid stimulates the release of ACTH (adrenocorticotropic hormone), which triggers adrenal steroid secretion and multifarious physiologic stress responses. In sum, AVP responds to sequelae of water loss and elicits a module of responses, including fluid retention, vasoconstriction with blood pressure maintenance, and mechanisms of the physiological stress response (figure 6.1).

Consideration of specific environmental stimuli, neural mechanisms, and diverse physiological effects in greater detail may indicate the precise role of AVP in the economy of information flow. AVP is synthesized in neurons of the supraoptic and paraventricular nuclei in the hypothalamus (figure 6.2). The neurons project to the posterior pituitary, where terminals release the octapeptide in response to appropriate stimuli. Total body water loss may result from a wide variety of conditions, including hemmorhage, liver disease, and passive dehydration. Water loss in turn may lead to reduced intravascular volume and increased plasma osmotic pressure (increased concentration), the proximate causes of AVP secretion. Reduced intravascular

SECRETION OF AVP

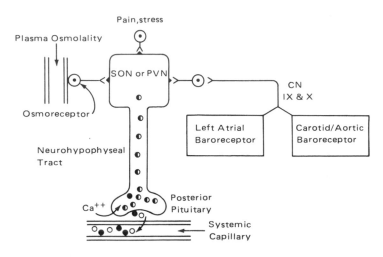

Figure 6.2
Anatomy of AVP secretion.
SON = supraoptic neuron; PVN = paraventricular neuron. (After Andreoli 1982)

volume tends to decrease blood pressure, which stimulates low pressure baroreceptors, or stretch receptors, located in the cardiovascular system. Baroreceptors, in the left atrium and aortic arch and at the carotid bifurcation, are excited by reduced pressure and convey impulses via the glossopharyngeal and vagus cranial nerves to the hypothalamus. Increased impulse activity liberates AVP from pituitary nerve terminals.

Increased plasma concentration (osmolality) stimulates osmoreceptors in the hypothalamus, also resulting in AVP secretion. Osmoreceptors are so exquisitely sensitive that even a 1 percent increase in plasma osmolality elicits AVP secretion. (Pain and stress also stimulate AVP secretion, although precise neural pathways and mechanisms have yet to be defined.)

In summary, a cluster of related physiological states stimulates the secretion of a single neuroeffector molecule through the excitation of highly specialized receptors. Such apparently diverse abnormalities as acute hemorrhage, liver disease with reduced vascular volume, or dehydration caused by water deprivation lead to the module of physiological responses mediated by AVP. Stimulation of baroreceptors and osmoreceptors ultimately results in the concerted stimulation of kidney, vascular smooth muscle, intestine, and pituitary through the mediation of AVP. Information flows from physiological state to specific neural receptors to the neuroeffector communicative molecule, AVP, and back to physiological state.

AVP elicits associated responses by acting directly on structures widely distributed in the body. The molecule binds to specific receptors on kidney tubule cells and vascular smooth muscle cells, and it interacts with pituitary and intestinal cells. Consequently the physiological AVP module results from the stimulation of geographically and functionally diverse cellular populations. That is, modular function is not simply localized to a geographically discrete area in the body. Rather, modularity derives from the concerted action of cells and systems throughout the organism.

AVP exhibits a certain inflexibility in the conversion of environmental information into the physiologic-behavioral module. Characteristically, stimulation of any single class of relevant receptors elicits the full panoply of AVP responses. For example, excitation of osmoreceptors, which monitor fluid balance governed by the kidney, results in cardiovascular changes and ACTH release, as well as alteration of kidney function. That is, an abormality of osmolality, a kidney-regulated state, elicits diverse cardiovascular, endocrine, and renal responses virtually indiscriminately. Similarly, stimulation of baroreceptors, osmoreceptors, or pain receptors individually yields the complete array of AVP actions. Since all the actions are incorporated in the single AVP molecule, fine-tuned controllability of output is lacking. However, these very structure-function relationships allow the neuroendocrine system to construct a multifaceted, integrated physiologic response from a stimulus fragment. In this and analogous instances, the biological system is "hard-wired" to execute complex modular repertoires in response to partial or fragmentary stimuli. The potential for more precise, and plastic, translation of specific stimuli into specific responses is present in true polyproteins, considered below.

Different responsive cells respond differently to AVP, leading, however, to a unified, integrated physiological response at the level of whole organism. **Stated differently, unity of the module emerges at the level of systems integration.** For example, epithelial cells located in different kidney tubules respond differently. In the collecting duct, AVP increases cellular permeability to water. In contrast, in renal medullary tubules, active sodium chloride transport is enhanced. However, these different responses at the cellular level result in an integrated response at the kidney level: the formation of concentrated urine with preservation of body water. At a higher level of integration, the conjunction of renal and vascular responses to AVP tends to preserve body water and cardiovascular hydrodynamics in the face of water loss. **The issues of levels of function and integration, and the emergence of "new" functions at higher levels, are even relevant to the physiology of the simple effector molecule, AVP.** Conversely, the integrated module governed by AVP is composed of levels of component parts at the multisystem, system, organ, cellular, and molecular levels. Mechanisms at different levels interact such that information flow is multidirectional, a phenomenon examined in detail in succeeding chapters.

With this introductory discussion as background, we proceed to consideration of true polyproteins, which contain multiple individual effector molecules, each coding for different actions.

Polyproteins and Opiate Peptides: POMC

Polyproteins participate in even more complicated physiological-behavioral repertoires. Proopiomelanocortin (POMC) is a prominent member of the class of known polyproteins (figure 6.3; for review, see Akil et al. 1984). ACTH, endorphin, and MSHs (melanocyte stimulating hormones) are released from the parent POMC molecule in the anterior pituitary in response to environmental stress. The peptides are also produced in the brain proper, in the arcuate nucleus of the mediobasal hypothalamus, and in the nucleus of the solitary tract. In turn, each peptide product exerts different actions. In concert, these actions constitute a physiological-behavioral module. ACTH stimulates adrenocortical cells to increase synthesis and release glucocorticoid hormones. The steroids exert a variety of effects, including enhanced glucose utilization, and the induction of a wide variety of enzymes involved in metabolic mobilization for the stress response. For example, glucocorticoids induce the catecholamine biosynthetic enzymes, tyrosine hydroxylase, dopamine-β-hydroxylase and phenylethanolamine-N-methytransferase, thereby increasing norepinephrine and epinephrine in sympathetics and adrenal. Consequently, ACTH, derived from POMC, indirectly stimulates somatic tissues and the sympathoadrenal axis, in one phase of the POMC module. The sympathoadrenal system directly participates in the fight-or-flight behavioral repertoire. Gamma-MSH, which is derived from the N-terminus of POMC, potentiates the steroidogenic actions of ACTH, thereby acting in a reinforcing mode (for review, see Herbert et al. 1984).

Endorphins released from POMC appear to mediate stress-induced analgesia, in which environmental emergency increases the threshold and tolerance for pain (for review, see Akil et al. 1984). In this well-

A: POMC

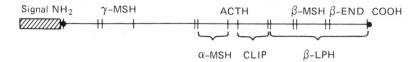

Signal NH₂ | γ-MSH | ACTH | β-MSH β-END COOH

α-MSH CLIP β-LPH

B: Pro-ENKEPHALIN

Leu-ENK

Met-ENK   Met-ENK

(Arg-Gly-Leu)   (Arg-Phe)

Signal NH₂   1 2   3   4   5   6   7 COOH

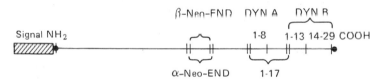

Peptide E

C: Pro-DYNORPHIN

β-Neo-END   DYN A   DYN B

Signal NH₂   1-8   1-13 14-29 COOH

α-Neo-END   1-17

Figure 6.3
Schematic representation of the protein precursor structures of the three opioid peptide families. Double vertical lines depict di-basic amino acid cleavage sites. (After Akil et al. 1984)

recognized though remarkable physiological-behavioral complex, emergent environmental events, such as life-threatening situations, radically alter pain perception processes. The threshold for stimulation of peripheral pain receptors actually increases. In parallel, central pain perception mechanisms are rendered less sensitive. Consequently endorphins allow the individual to mobilize, attack, defend, or escape in the face of physical insult and injury that would otherwise disable. The performance of heroic acts under debilitating fire reflects, in part, endorphin analgesia. By altering pain reception and perception, endorphins permit the translation of ACTH metabolic mobilization into appropriate, potentially life-saving behavior.

Study of pain modification by POMC substituents has revealed complex relations among the polyprotein components. The POMC products act synergistically in the control of pain. ACTH evokes analgesia in the central grey through nonopiate receptors (Walker et al. 1980a and 1980b). Moreover, ACTH-like agents and endorphin are additive analgesics, and gamma-MSH, which is inactive alone, potentiates ACTH analgesia. Although each polyprotein product exerts unique actions, it is apparent that the components also participate in common, mutually reinforcing actions. Remarkably, the individual peptides modulate pain perception through different, as well as common, physiological mechanisms. ACTH and endorphin, for example, engage different receptors and neural systems to modify the same sensory complex, pain. The parent polyprotein encodes a fascinating logic that appears to lie at the heart of this modular organization.

Opiate peptides also regulate cardiovascular function, specifically governing blood pressure through a number of mechanisms (see Akil et al. 1984 for review). However, no simple generalizations have yet emerged in this new area. Opiates may be pressor or depressor, depending on conditions and route of administration.

To summarize, in response to stressful situations, the components of POMC induce a complex, self-reinforcing, stereotyped battery of actions. These actions complement the plastic sympathoadrenal and brain coeruleal transmitter changes already described to elicit adaptive behavioral responses.

Other Opiate Polyproteins

POMC is but one of three different endogenous opiate polyproteins. The others—proenkephalin (Comb et al. 1982; Gubler et al. 1981; Hughes et al. 1975; Kimura et al. 1980; Mizuno et al. 1980; Noda et al. 1982a, 1982b) and prodynorphin (Fischli et al. 1982; Goldstein et al. 1979, 1981; Kakidani et al. 1982; Kangawa et al. 1981)—are also synthesized as precursor molecules that release several bioactive components upon processing (figure 6.4). The different polyproteins are differentially distributed in multiple neuronal populations, and functional interrelationships have yet to be elucidated. Nevertheless, the potential for diversity and complexity is already evident. For example, the peptide products elaborated by any neuronal population are dependent on cellular orchestration of the enzymes that process precursor and products. The entire process is cell specific and differs for different neurons. The precursor polyprotein is cleaved differently in different populations, leading to the production of unique biologic activities. Further, posttranslational processing, which modifies a product after translation of mRNA into protein, differs with neuronal type. Thus, the cleavage products are subject to acetylation, amidation, phosphorylation, glycosylation, and methylation in a cell-specific manner. Each modification alters biologic activity in a cell-specific fashion and determines ratios of final peptides. In turn, different peptides interact with different receptors, eliciting different biologic effects. It is abundantly clear that the particular physiological-behavioral module activated by a polyprotein is not simply determined by the genetic code for the precursor. In fact, the role of the environment and of extracellular, epigenetic factors in the regulation of polyprotein processing and module modification is the subject of intense study.

Despite such confusing diversity, commonalities of structure and function are discernible. Opiate functions are dependent on the enkephalin structure, which is present in the proenkephalin polyprotein as methionine-enkephalin and leucine enkephalin (figures 6.3 and 6.4). All other opiate peptides are simply C terminal extensions of leu- or met-enkephalin. For example, beta-endorphin is a 26 amino acid, C terminal extension of met-enk (see Herbert et al. 1984 for review), and dynorphin is a 12 amino acid extension of leu-enk. Consequently, all known endogenous opiate activities, whether nociceptive or cardiovascular, regardless of parent polyprotein or neural system localization, are based on a common chemical structure. That structure is encoded by the genome, and our search for the origins of associated behaviors, the origins of modularity, now requires knowledge of the genomic organization underlying polyprotein elaboration.

Genomic Organization of Polyproteins

How are polyproteins, and associated behaviors, encoded at the level of the genome? In fact, are behavioral modules actually represented in genes? Does genomic organization govern forms of expression of behavioral modules? Does gene structure determine which environ-

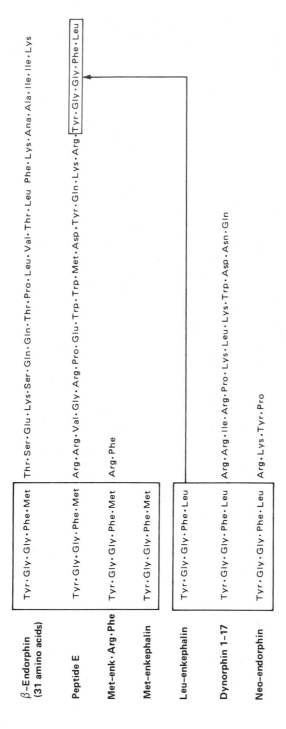

Figure 6.4
Structure of the opioid peptides indicating common functional enkephalin sequences. Twenty-five of the 31 amino acids of β-endorphin are shown. (From Herbert et al. 1984)

mental stimuli elicit a behavioral repertoire? In brief, does genomic organization dictate environment-behavior relations and the very existence of modular organization?

Synthesis of opioid polyproteins is directed by at least three different genes. One gene codes for proenkephalin, which contains six met-enk and one leu-enk sequence (for reviews see Herbert et al. 1984; Akil et al. 1984). Another gene codes for POMC, which contains beta-endorphin, ACTH, and alpha-, beta- and gamma-MSH. A third gene encodes prodynorphin, the precursor for dynorphin and neoendorphins. Since each polyprotein contains different combinations of neuroactive peptides and since multiple opioid receptor subtypes mediate different physiologic-behavioral effects, different genes code for distinct, but often overlapping, behavioral modules.

Does knowledge of the gene structures provide information regarding regulation of behavioral expression and insight into the molecular organization of behavior? Can we identify features of the genome that are central to the transduction from environment to behavior, from experience to biology? Opiates have been implicated in euphoria, relief of the subjective experience of pain, and addictive behavior. Can we define specific genomic structures and processes that underlie these subjective states? Even a few tentative steps would have a major impact on our understanding of mind, emotion, and cognition.

Initially we can focus on general characteristics of organization of the opioid polyprotein genome. Is modularity encoded in genes? Can we detect evolutionary relationships among behaviorally similar putative modules? In fact, structural similarity of the opioid polyproteins suggests that the peptides are closely related phylogenetically. The close relationship should be detectable in the structure of genes encoding the peptides. Eukaryotic genes contain coding regions, termed exons, separated by the noncoding introns. The arrangement of these regions may provide insight into gene regulation and organization of behavior. Indeed, striking similarities have already been discovered between the POMC and proenkephalin genes. All of the known biologically active peptides derived from proenkephalin and POMC are encoded within a single large exon (for review, see Herbert et al. 1984). More specifically, both genes contain large exons that code for more than 80 percent of the protein (figure 6.5). A large intron on the side of the exon separates it from the exon that encodes the so-called signal sequence of each polyprotein. These observations define commonalities in the organization of genes that determine organization of behavior. Different opiate polyprotein genes, which code for clusters of related behaviors, are similarly organized. It is apparent that modules of associated behaviors are encoded in the genome. Modularity of

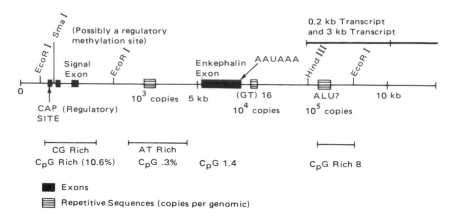

Figure 6.5
Organization of the human proenkephalin gene. The left-hand side represents the 5′ end. Exons are indicated by boxes. Sites digested by restriction endonucleases EcoRI, SmaI, and HindIII are indicated. (From Herbert et al. 1984)

neuroeffector mechanisms is an inherited trait. **The association of bioactive sequences in a single gene results in the obligatory association of encoded behaviors and the existence of modularity itself.**

Phylogenetic parallels are implied. The structural similarities between the opioid genes indicate a close evolutionary relationship between genes, and between the behaviors subserved (Herbert et al. 1984). The POMC and proenkephalin genes apparently are derived from a common primordial gene from which they diverged. Evolution from the progenitor gene may have occurred through duplication of DNA sequences, through point mutation, or through translocation of a portion of the gene. Regardless of specific mechanism, it is apparent that the evolution of modules involving analgesia and euphoria, for example, may now be defined at the behavioral and molecular levels simultaneously. Specific molecular mechanisms responsible for the taxonomy of related behaviors may now be delineated, and behaviors and underlying molecular mechanisms may be followed through phyletic lineages. Moreover, the genesis of related behavioral modules, derived from the action of related genes such as POMC and proenkephalin, is accessible to detailed analysis.

Study of gene structure may also help define environment-behavior relations by indicating potential sites of regulation by extracellular stimuli. Analysis of human DNA (by Southern blot) has indicated only a single human proenkephalin gene (Comb et al. 1983). Structural analysis of the gene and its flanking regions has been performed. One particularly striking structural characteristic may provide clues to the regulation of gene expression and, consequently, behavior. Both the POMC and proenkephalin genes exhibit markedly asymmetric distributions of guanine (G) and cytosine (C) residues (Herbert et al. 1984). CpG sequences cluster in the 5' and 3' untranslated regions of the genes. This observation is of extreme interest since methylation of C residues in this sequence has been implicated in the ontogenetic regulation of gene expression. Transcription of a gene appears to vary inversely as the degree of methylation of C bases in the CpG sequence (Felsenfeld and McGhee 1982). It may now be possible to determine whether methylation and demethylation regulate readout of these different polyprotein genes, thereby governing appropriate behavioral modules. In turn, this is a potentially important site for environmental regulation. For example, specific environmental stimuli may selectively methylate or demethylate the gene through action on transmethylase enzymes. It may now be possible to move from environmental stimulus to gene expression to behavioral repertoire in a logical, causal sequence.

One approach to the role of methylation in polyprotein gene expression is to examine the proenkephalin gene in different tissues. Since expression is tissue specific, the level of cytosine methylation may be correlated with expression. DNA was isolated from a number of human tissues—some, such as adrenal, that express enkephalin, and some, such as leukocytes, that do not. Specific CpG sites that are less methylated have been discovered in DNA from the adrenal. Tissues that do not express the gene products have higher levels of methylation (Herbert et al. 1984).

Recombinant DNA techniques were used to determine whether the specific demethlylated sites were, in fact, involved in the regulation of expresson. One hint might derive from the location of the sites. Analysis indicated that one of the demethylated CpG sites is just 3' to the site for initiation of transcription (readout or gene expression), the cap site (Herbert et al. 1984). There is a high probability that demethylation of this site does regulate expression. Experiments are now in progress to alter the structure of the methylation sites directly and define effects on the level of expression (see Herbert et al. 1984 for details). Moreover, it is now possible to determine whether environmental stimuli or signals specifically alter methylation of the gene, and thereby regulate expression of the behavioral module.

The Polyprotein Module in Invertebrates

A number of relatively simple, primitive animals have been used to study behavior and underlying molecular and electrophysiologic mechanisms. The work of Kandel and colleagues on the sea snail (Kandel and Schwartz 1982) is beginning to place such behavioral phenomena as habituation, dishabituation, and sensitization on a firm molecular footing (see Kandel 1976). Experiments with the sea snail have also led to the realization that the polyprotein strategy is employed in the regulation of behavior by this relatively primitive marine mollusc.

Egg-laying behavior in the sea snail is a stereotyped, yet complex, behavioral module regulated by a family of neuropeptides (for review, see Scheller et al. 1983b). The atrial gland secretes the A and B peptides, which depolarize two groups of electrically coupled neurons in the abdominal ganglion. These ganglion "bag cells" in turn discharge and secrete multiple peptides, including the critical egg-laying hormone (ELH). The peptides enter a highly vascularized sheath that surrounds the ganglion and are transported to proximate and distant targets. The peptides exert a number of effects. They alter the electrical excitability of central neurons and simultaneously stimulate distant targets, including the ovotestis, via the circulation. Consequently the complex egg-laying behavioral module results from the synchronized transmitter, hormonal, and modulatory actions of these neuropeptides. In summary, the atrial gland releases the A and B peptides, which elicit bag cell firing, the release of ELH and associated peptides with consequent CNS and ovotestis stimulation, and performance of the egg-laying behavioral repertoire. Can we analyze the genomic basis of this behavioral module and determine whether regulatory features are shared with the opioid peptide family already discussed?

The neuropeptides that govern egg-laying behavior and associated physiology are encoded by a relatively small gene family (Scheller et al. 1982, 1983a, 1983b). The homologous genes include those for ELH and peptide B, which are linked, and the gene for peptide A. The gene family is expressed by the bag cells, the atrial gland, and a network of interneurons widely distributed in the CNS. Different members of the gene family are expressed in different tissues; for example, bag cells predominantly express ELH, and the atrial gland contains peptide A and B.

Each gene in the family codes for a different polyprotein composed of the neuroactive peptides flanked by proteolytic cleavage sites. Proteolysis at these specific sites results in liberation of the individual, biologically active products. Although the genes exhibit greater than 90 percent homology at the DNA level, small differences in sequence have led to significant alteration in specific amino acids that regulate processing of the polyproteins. Consequently, while all the polyproteins apparently contain A and B peptides and ELH, each precursor releases a different peptide upon processing. In summary, entirely different peptides may be released from highly homologous polyproteins encoded by closely related genes. The biologic strategy, then, is analogous to that described for the opioid peptides. Distinct behavioral modules are encoded by closely related genes. Differential processing at the level of the polyprotein can lead to remarkable molecular and behavioral diversity.

Organization of the prototypical ELH gene has emerged from extensive work involving the use of cDNA and genomic clones, restriction mapping, gene sequencing, and hybridization studies (Mahon et al. 1985). Many facets of the gene structure are typical of eukaryotic genes and emphasize that genes controlling behavior are not qualitatively different from those governing other cell functions. For example, the ELH gene consists of three exons, separated by a single intron. Characteristically, consensus sequences that initiate transcription in eukaryotes—the so-called TATA and CAAT boxes—are located upstream from exon 1. Additional sequences that regulate processing of messenger RNA in all eukaryotes have been identified. Moreover, sequence homology among different genes of the ELH family markedly decreases upstream from the initiation sequences, a locus that governs tissue-specific expression in other systems. Changes in these DNA sequences may be critical in the evolution of tissue-specific gene expression, paralleling structural differences noted in the growth hormone gene family.

The emerging picture of the ELH family incorporates plasticity in the face of genome-encoded behavior. Tissue-specific polyprotein processing regulated by specific environmental stimuli leads to flexibility of module form and expression. Consequently, sexual behavior in the sea snail exhibits the potential for flexibility and stereotypy simultaneously. We shall certainly want to examine the molecular, cellular, and systems basis for such potential in mammalian forms as well.

Some General Considerations

We have now examined several prominent examples of the polyprotein strategy, and a number of principles have emerged. Most generally, it is possible to move from gene to message, protein product, and behavior in a comprehensible causal manner, although a myriad of mechanistic details remain to be characterized. Whether considering vasopressin, opioid peptides, or ELH, the continuity from molecule to physiologic effects and behavior is unmistakable. While this appears obvious and almost trivial after our detailed discussions, the theoretical and practical implications could scarcely be more important. From a practical point of view, these realizations dictate experimental strategies that integrate the study of effector molecules and behavior. Further, disordered behavior and disease may be analyzed at a definable sequence of loci from gene to molecular signals to behavior, allowing definition of pathogenesis and evolution of new therapeutic approaches.

From a theoretical viewpoint, our discussions define precise symbols in the mind-brain system and unambiguously begin to characterize interrelationships. Conversely, there is no need to posit the existence of entirely different domains to explain behavior and mentation. Nevertheless, although functions can be described reasonably crisply, it is apparent that there is no comfortable, sharp divide between biology and behavior. Behavior or mental state represents a complex of molecular-physiological interactions occurring in and among specific neural subsystems. This bare-bones description belies formidable complexities. However, the complexities lie within the very functions and relationships that we have been defining. But haven't we simply ignored the role of network theory and processing? On the contrary, we are defining the very units, the foundation, upon which networks and local systems processing are built. No network theory that does not consider the constraints imposed at the molecular and behavioral levels can be considered complete.

The salient point is that neurobiology of mental function derives from cellular biology itself. We may look to mechanisms of cellular biology to discern the units of cognitive function, the roots of mentation, an issue to which we return.

Finally, consideration of the polyprotein strategy has defined modular organization of behavior at the molecular level. Is modularity of human brain function explicable in molecular terms as well? What are the contributions of the molecular, cellular, and systems domains to modularity of human cognitive function, if any?

Chapter 7

Molecules and Systems: Trophic Interactions

---

*Systems in Context—Trophic Molecules and Systems—Nerve Growth
Factor, Peripheral Systems, and Function—Nerve Growth Factor and
Systems Relations—The Nerve Growth Factor Molecule—Trophic
Interactions in the Brain—Nerve Growth Factor, Acetylcholine, and
Memory*

While the organization of molecular signals contributes to the existence of modularity, organization of the brain into systems constitutes
a complementary precondition. Indeed, while signals comprise units
of organization in one domain, neural subsystems are the larger functional units within which the molecules act. Compartmentalization in
subsystems, each subserving discrete behavioral and physiologic functions, endows behavior, emotionality, and cognition with characteristic qualities. What mechanisms are responsible for the particular
pattern of systems organization of the brain? How are systems built,
and how are they maintained? Do specific cellular and even molecular
mechanisms contribute to systems construction, function, and organization? Do molecular signals build and maintain the very systems
in which signals function?

Increasing evidence suggests that multiple classes of molecules contribute to systems organization. For example, cell adhesion molecules
and surface adhesion molecules help guide growing nerve processes
to appropriate targets, contributing to the formation of functional
connections (for review, see Rutishauser and Jessell 1988; Edelman
1988). On the other hand, trophic molecules (troph = nutrition) appear
to play a central system-specific role in the genesis, maintenance, and
function of subsystems (for an overview, see Purves 1988). We employ
trophic functions as models to understand signal-system relations and
the nature of systems organization.

Trophic molecules regulate manifold processes necessary for the
development, maintenance, and normal function of specific, respon-

sive pathways. The survival of receptive neurons during development is dependent on exposure to the appropriate trophic molecule(s). Evidence derived from in vitro studies suggests that trophic factors also help guide (tropic function) growing nerve processes to appropriate targets, thereby fostering the formation of specific synaptic connections. Connectivity itself appears to be regulated by trophic molecules, since appropriate targets elaborate the specific factor selectively required by innervating neurons. The factors are necessary for maintenance and normal pathway function during maturity, suggesting that trophism functions throughout life. Trophic factors stimulate transmitter function in receptive neurons, suggesting that transmission itself may be under trophic control. Finally, different neuronal populations that innervate the same target may compete for common target trophic factors. Consequently, co-innervating populations may communicate through unconventional means.

In sum, in the now-traditional model, neurons compete for target-elaborated trophic molecules (figure 7.1). Those neurons that make successful connections gain access to sustaining trophic factor and

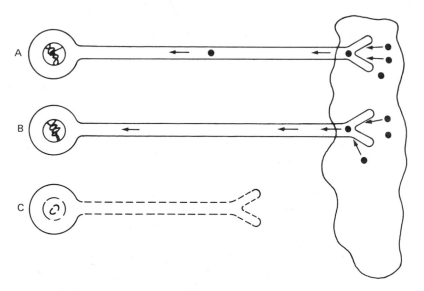

Figure 7.1
Traditional model of trophic interactions: Target regulation, survival, and competition. Targets elaborate trophic factors that interact with those neurons that have successfully innervated the target, thereby ensuring neuronal survival. The lowest neuron, which has failed to innervate the target, is deprived of sustaining target trophic factor and consequently dies.

survive and function; neurons failing to make appropriate connections are deprived of factor and die. An ongoing supply of factor is necessary for normal system function throughout life. It is apparent that trophic molecules contribute to the organization of systems and the very existence of neural subsystems. With this general background, we examine the prototypical trophic molecule, nerve growth factor (NGF). Initially we examine NGF in the relatively simple peripheral nervous system to discern the relationship of trophic molecule, system, and physiological-behavioral function.

NGF, Peripheral Systems, and Function

NGF is the most completely delineated trophic factor. Early work by Levi-Montalcini, Hamburger, and colleagues indicated that NGF is necessary for the survival and development of sympathetic and sensory neurons in avian and mammalian species (figure 7.2; for historical overview, see Levi-Montalcini and Angeletti 1968; Hamburger et al. 1949, 1981; Bradshaw 1978). Moreover, after extensive search lasting decades, increasing evidence indicates that the trophic agent plays a critical role in brain systems function. I briefly summarize work performed in the periphery to illustrate the role of trophic interactions in the development, maintenance, and function of connectivity.

In the nervous system, as in most organ systems, cells are vastly overproduced during early ontogeny, with subsequent death of up to 80 percent in many populations (Glucksman 1951; Cowan et al. 1984). Treatment with NGF markedly enhances sensory and sympathetic survival, and anti-NGF antiserum (anti-NGF) prevents survival through NGF deprivation (Levi-Montalcini and Angeletti 1968). Specific high-affinity and low-affinity receptors have been identified on the cell membranes of receptive populations (Sutter et al. 1984). NGF is elaborated by target cells that are innervated by sensory and sympathetic neurons in the periphery (Hendry et al. 1974a and 1974b; Korsching and Thoenen 1983; Ebendal et al. 1983; Shelton and Reichardt 1984). Consequently, appropriate innervation of a target by sensory or sympathetic neurons ensures that the neurons will be exposed to the required trophic agent, thereby ensuring neuronal survival and pathway development and maintenance. NGF synthesized and released by targets is taken up by responsive neurons and transported in a retrograde fashion from terminals to cell body (figure 7.1; Hendry et al. 1974a,1974b; Stockel et al. 1975a, 1975b; Hendry 1977; Johnson et al. 1978; Brunso-Bechtold and Hamburger 1979). However, the precise site of action of NGF in the neuron remains to be identified.

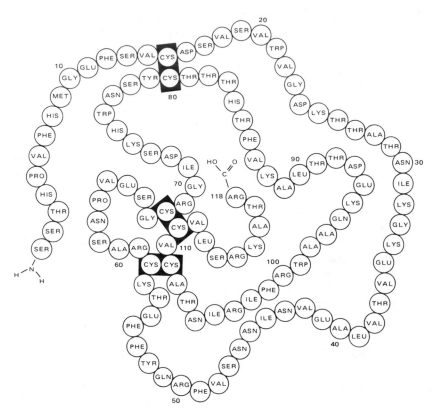

Figure 7.2
The β-subunit of NGF. This is a schematic representation of a single chain of the biologically active portion of the NGF molecule. (From Angeletti and Bradshaw 1971)

In summary, sensory and sympathetic neurons are overproduced during development, and competition for NGF determines which neurons will survive and which, through deprivation, will die. Results of this competition define neural systems, determining lines of communication through connectivity.

NGF is actually misnamed since it also functions during maturity to maintain connections between receptive neurons and NGF-producing target cells. For example, interruption of the retrograde transport of NGF in the adult or treatment of adults with anti-NGF results in sympathetic dysfunction and compromised sympathetic-target communication (Bjerre et al. 1975a, 1975b; Kessler and Black 1979). Consequently trophic function maintains gross structural integrity of neural systems during maturity; NGF appears to be necessary for normal systems function throughout life.

In addition to serving a maintenance role, NGF appears to regulate systems function dynamically. For example, NGF increases the levels of transmitters localized to receptive neurons, presumably enhancing transmission (for example, see Bjerre et al. 1975a). The trophic molecule increases catecholamine biosynthetic enzymes (Thoenen et al. 1971) and norepinephrine in sympathetics (Bjerre et al. 1975a) and increases substance P, the peptide transmitter, in sensory neurons (Kessler and Black 1980). In sum, NGF regulates physical circuit connectivity and simultaneously governs communication through the elaboration of presynaptic transmitter. Trophic molecules, connectivity and transmitters, and gross structure and function are intimately related.

By regulating specific systems, that serve discrete behaviors, NGF indirectly contributes to specific behavioral repertoires. For example, NGF is clearly required for development and normal function of the system that governs the fight-or-flight response. Trophic molecules, then, contribute to the molar organization of behavior and to systems development and function that participate in modular organization.

NGF and Systems Relations

In addition to the roles played by the trophic factor in communication within a system, NGF exerts more subtle, indirect effects on systems interactions. Since sympathetic and sensory systems require NGF for normal development and function and since the systems innervate common targets in many instances, competitive interactions might be anticipated (figure 7.1). Recent experiments substantiate this expectation: co-innervating sympathetic and sensory neurons compete for target-elaborated NGF (Kessler et al. 1983b). For example, extirpation of the sympathetic innervation to a target results in increased measures of sensory innervation. This increase is reversed by artificial implantation of sympathetics. Moreover, administration of NGF reproduces the effects of sympathetic ablation, increasing sensory innervation. Conversely, local anti-NGF (antiserum) treatment decreases sensory innervation, suggesting that target-derived NGF normally regulates sensory innervation. Finally, anti-NGF treatment reverses the effects of sympathetic removal, suggesting that sympathetic and sensory terminals compete for target NGF.

In summary, functionally and anatomically distinct, co-innervating neural populations compete for a common, target-derived trophic factor. The outcome of that competition determines cell survival, relative pathway size, and patterns of connectivity. Since NGF is necessary throughout life, ongoing competition may regulate pathway relations during maturity, as well as development. In a sense, by competing for a common trophic factor, co-innervating neurons communicate in an indirect fashion. Thus, NGF both regulates individual systems and influences the pattern of systems relations.

Characteristics of the NGF Molecule

What mechanisms allow trophic molecules to build functional systems? How is the information in NGF converted to a functioning sympathetic system, subserving fight or flight, or to a sensory system, processing pain and touch? What characteristics of the NGF molecule are necessary for biologic activity? How is synthesis regulated, and how is the NGF molecule processed? Finally, how is systems specificity conferred such that only a restricted set responds to NGF? Although our knowledge is rudimentary, general outlines are beginning to emerge.

The accepted view envisages what may be termed a minimal trophic unit (figure 7.1). **Postsynaptic targets** elaborate **trophic factor,** which interacts with **receptors** on specific **presynaptic neurons** (for review, see Purves 1988). Interaction with biologically active receptor results in internalization of the NGF-receptor complex, retrograde transport to cell body, and the panoply of actions leading to neuron survival, system formation, and regulation of transmission. What is the nature of the NGF molecule and its receptor?

NGF biologic activity is associated with the beta subunit, a dimer of covalently linked, identical polypeptide chains, each containing 118 amino acids of defined sequence (figure 7.2; Greene and Shooter 1980; Angeletti and Bradshaw 1971; Angeletti et al. 1973a, 1973b; Bradshaw 1978). The beta subunit is contained in a multisubunit, storage complex, 7s NGF, consisting of an alpha2-gamma2-beta1 composition, stabilized by zinc ions. Based on these data, it might be anticipated that biologic activity requires release of the beta subunit from the parent complex. How is this processing accomplished?

The gamma subunit is an arginine esteropeptidase enzyme that releases the active beta subunit, allowing interaction with receptor and expression of biologic effects. The alpha subunit is an acidic protein, and interactions among the subunits and zinc ions stabilize the complex. However, the precise mechanisms underlying stabilization and alternative beta subunit release remain to be elucidated. It is not clear, for example, whether 7s processing even represents an important regulatory locus where environmental influences may intervene. Similarly, the regulation of beta subunit synthesis is largely uncharted.

NGF is synthesized by targets, and the level of encoding mRNA correlates with density of innervation by specific responsive neurons (Shelton and Reichardt 1984). It is unclear, however, whether synthesis is specifically regulated by epigenetic factors. Innervating neurons do not appear to govern synthesis by target. In fact, targets continue to synthesize and release trophic factor after denervation (see, for example, Ebendal et al. 1980). Moreover, the factors responsible for initial expression of the NGF gene by targets remain to be elucidated.

Although the regulation of NGF synthesis remains an open question, the factors that govern specificity of responsiveness are somewhat clearer. Neurons are specifically responsive by virtue of expressing NGF receptors. Low-affinity ($K_d=10^{-9}M$) and high-affinity ($K_d=10^{-11}M$) forms have been identified (for review, see Greene and Shooter, 1980). Biologic activity appears to be mediated by binding to the high-affinity receptor. The relationship between low- and high-affinity receptors is still obscure. There is only a single NGF receptor gene, and only a single mRNA has been isolated (Chao et al. 1986). Consequently the two receptor forms are the product of a single gene. However, factors influencing potential receptor interconversion are undefined, although this obviously constitutes a critical issue in understanding systems formation by NGF. Moreover, the intrinsic or extrinsic factors that induce specific populations to elaborate NGF receptors are undefined.

Trophic Interactions in the Brain

In the periphery, NGF participates in the development and function of systems subserving fight or flight and the reception of sensory stimuli. Consequently trophic interactions in the peripheral system are important determinants of the organization of well-circumscribed behavioral repertoires. Recent work now indicates that NGF functions in an analogous fashion in the brain. However, this realization emerged only after decades of false starts and confusing leads. In fact, until recently, prevailing wisdom held that NGF played no role in brain function. This erroneous conclusion was based on work predicated on a tacit, unwarranted assumption. It might be useful to digress briefly and describe the nature of this assumption since the brain sciences, in their complexity, invite just this type of error.

NGF elicits striking increases in norepinephrine (NE) in sympathetic neurons, in addition to regulating sympathetic growth and the formation of connections. Based on these dramatic observations, workers throughout the world examined catecholaminergic neurons in the brain to determine whether NGF regulated the function of these cells. After numerous conflicting studies and confusing suggestions, general agreement emerged: central NE neurons were not responsive to NGF and certainly not dependent on the trophic protein for survival, development, or the formation of connections. It was concluded that NGF had no central actions.

In retrospect, there had been no reason to assume that NGF was a trophic agent for catecholaminergic neurons exclusively. Indeed, as the putative peptide transmitters were identified in sensory and sympathetic populations, it became apparent that NGF also increased these transmitters. More important, there was no reason to perpetuate the tacit assumption that NGF was transmitter specific. Freed of this debilitating assumption, we now examine the role of NGF in regulating **non**catecholaminergic systems and functions in the brain.

Many processes involved in systems formation in the periphery also occur in brain, suggesting that comparable trophic interactions might underlie central pattern formation. For example, neurons are markedly overproduced in brain as in the periphery; central neurons and systems also compete for synaptic sites; increasing evidence indicates that central neurons that contact appropriate targets survive, while unconnected neurons die, consistent with target trophic effects (for review see Cowan et al. 1984). What specific systems, and resultant behavioral functions, appear to be regulated by NGF, the prototypical trophic molecule?

Cholinergic neurons, which are located in the basal forebrain and project widely to the cerebral cortex, have recently been the focus of intense interest (figure 7.3; Mesulam 1989; Mesulam and Geula 1988; Mesulam et al. 1984, 1986). This prominent group of nuclei subserves critical cognitive functions and degenerates in Alzheimer's disease (Whitehouse et al. 1982). In addition, neurons in this population respond to NGF and may be dependent on the factor for normal devel-

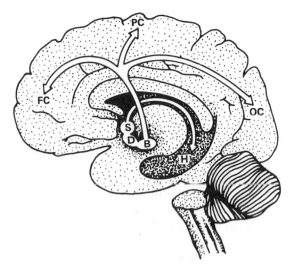

Figure 7.3
NGF and basal forebrain: Schematic representation of the basal forebrain–cortical cholinergic system. The cholinergic cell bodies of the basal forebrain are located in the
nucleus basalis of Meynert (B), the diagonal band of Broca (D), and the medial septal
nucleus (S). All neurons send projection axons to innervate the cerebral cortex, including
frontal (FC), parietal (PC), and occipital (OC) areas, as well as the hippocampal formation (H). (From Coyle et al. 1983)

opment and function (for review, see Whittemore and Seiger 1987).
Specific cognitive functions, trophic factor, and systems functions may
be fruitfully examined in the context of the basal forebrain-cortical
network.

In particular, we focus on the septo-hippocampal system, consisting
of neurons that project from the septal area of the basal forebrain to
the hippocampal cortex (figure 7.3). This system, and the hippocampus as a target, play a critical role in contextual-spatial memory. Extensive study by many workers, including O'Keefe and Nadel, Olton
and colleagues, McNaughton and colleagues, Eichenbaum, and others, has clearly established that the hippocampus encodes spatial
memory in the rat (for example, see O'Keefe and Nadel 1978; Berger
and Thompson 1978; Olton et al. 1979; Eichenbaum and Cohen 1988;
Eichenbaum et al. 1989; Olton 1989). Moreover, the hippocampus
codes for complex memory tasks in subhuman primates, as demonstrated by the elegant studies of Mishkin and colleagues (for review,
see Mishkin 1982), and is critical for mnemonic function in humans,
indicated by the classic work of Milner (1970) and the more recent
observations of Squire (1986).

Analysis of the rat model has been detailed, and is particularly germane, since this species has been employed most extensively to study brain NGF. Lesions of the hippocampus profoundly impair the rat's ability to store information concerning spatial relations in the environment. For example, the lesioned animal is unable to perform adequately on a radial arm maze, in search of food placed in novel arms on different trials after a training period (Olton et al. 1979). Septo-hippocampal lesions induce similar behavioral deficits. Moreover, the hippocampus codes for environmental relations more complicated than simple spatial relations. For example, direction of movement, attitude of the head with respect to body plane, and movement sequence all affect hippocampal neuron response. According to the dominant view, then, the hippocampus codes for environmental spatial relations in the context of the organism's experience and motor activity (Eichenbaum et al. 1989). Normal function of the septo-hippocampal system underlies this complex behavioral repertoire. Emerging studies suggest that the basal forebrain neurons, and their projections in the septo-hippocampal system, are responsive to NGF and dependent on the trophic protein for normal function. A brief summary of the mounting evidence may help define the relationship of behavior, neural system, trophic factor, and transmitter.

Complementary studies, performed in vivo and in vitro, indicate that NGF plays a critical role in the basal forebrain-hippocampal system. NGF protein and its mRNA have been detected in the rat hippocampus, indicating that the factor is synthesized within this target of the basal forebrain neurons (Large et al. 1986; Shelton and Reichardt 1986; Korsching et al. 1985). Moreover, NGF mRNA has been localized to target pyramidal and granule neurons in the hippocampus (Ayer-LeLievre et al. 1988). Conversely, NGF high-affinity receptor and its mRNA are present in the basal forebrain cholinergic neurons, indicating that the population is potentially responsive (Bernd et al. 1988; Buck et al. 1987). As expected, NGF is transported in a retrograde fashion from cortex terminals to perikarya in the basal forebrain (Schwab et al. 1979). Finally, exogenous NGF reportedly exerts a variety of actions on the basal forebrain neurons in vivo (Mobley et al. 1986). NGF increases the acetylcholine biosynthetic enzyme, choline acetyltransferase (CAT), specifically localized to these neurons (Gnahn et al. 1983; Hefti et al. 1985; Martinez et al. 1987). Moreover, administration of NGF prevents necrosis of these cells consequent to septo-hippocampal (fimbria-fornix) lesion (Hefti et al. 1986; Kromer et al. 1987; Williams et al. 1986). Most dramatic, NGF also reverses the behavioral deficit in spatial memory in aged rats (Gage et al. 1986).

Studies in culture of basal forebrain neurons suggest that NGF acts directly on these neurons, not indirectly by affecting other cells. Cholinergic neurons in culture exhibit specific high-affinity NGF receptors, and NGF increases CAT and acetylcholinesterase, specific indexes of cholinergic function (Bernd et al. 1988; Martinez et al. 1987). Moreover, NGF dramatically increases the number of CAT-positive neurons in culture, raising the possibility that NGF directly enhances cholinergic neuron survival. Finally, basal forebrain neurons express the NGF receptor gene in culture, definitively indicating that these cholinergic cells have the intrinsic capacity to elaborate specific receptors (Lu et al. 1989).

Are the effects of NGF specific and selective for the cholinergic basal forebrain-cortical system? In fact, the effects of NGF on forebrain neurons are blocked by anti-NGF antiserum, indicating marked specificity (Martinez et al. 1987). Moreover, molecules that are structurally similar to NGF fail to reproduce effects of the trophic factor. Conversely, NGF selectively affects the cholinergic population, since other basal forebrain neurons, such as those containing somatostatin or those containing substance P, are unaffected by the trophic factor. (Nevertheless, recent work does indicate that some noncholinergic neurons in the basal forebrain may also respond to NGF [Dreyfus et al. 1989].) Consequently, in the brain, as in the periphery, NGF specifically and selectively regulates well-circumscribed systems that subserve discrete behavioral modules.

A provisional model can be constructed by synthesizing insights derived from study of peripheral as well as central NGF. During development, the septal pathway, emanating from basal cholinergic neurons, makes synaptic contact with hippocampal neurons. NGF may act as a "guidance" factor, directly or indirectly orienting fibers toward the hippocampus, as has been suggested for peripheral neurons. Additionally, NGF elaborated by hippocampal neurons may ensure that those forebrain neurons that do make successful hippocampal contact survive, thereby developing the pathway. It is reasonable to assume that NGF is necessary for pathway maintenance during maturity, as in the periphery. Consequently, ongoing function of the NGF trophic unit is necessary for the storage of spatial memory during adulthood, as well as system formation during development. Communication among trophic molecules, exemplified by NGF-receptor interactions, constructs and maintains the capacity for spatial mnemonic function. Exercise of that capacity, however, depends on transmitter function. Consideration of transmitter function, in turn, emphasizes cholinergic system specificity for spatial memory function and organization of the brain into trophic-transmitter system units.

NGF, Acetylcholine, and Memory

Evidence from a variety of sources implicates cholinergic mechanisms in memory function, and in the septo-hippocampal system in particular. Administration of the cholinergic antagonist scopolamine to humans depresses memory function (see, for example, Drachman and Leavitt, 1974). Conversely, physostigmine, a cholinergic agonist, improves memory function. In parallel observations in monkeys, cholinergic agonists improve memory, and antagonists inhibit memory function (Bartus and Johnson 1976; Bartus 1978). Administration of cholinergic antagonists to rats reproduces the effects of septo-hippocampal surgical lesions in eliciting spatial memory dysfunction (Fukuchi et al. 1987; Meyers and Domino 1964; Douglas and Truncer 1976; Okaichi and Jarrard 1982; Wirsching et al. 1984; Westlind et al. 1981). Similarly, cholinergic agents predictably alter memory function after septo-hippocampal lesions (see Eckerman et al. 1980; Ksir et al. 1974). Hippocampal CAT activity is markedly reduced in Alzheimer's disease, a disorder in which memory deficits are a hallmark (Kuhar 1976; Bowen et al. 1981). Moreover, extensive degeneration of the basal forebrain cholinergic neurons is a prominent feature of this disease (Whitehouse et al. 1981, 1982; Coyle et al. 1983). In addition, a number of studies suggest that reduced cortical CAT accompanies memory deficits that occur during normal aging, although this is an area of lively debate (for review, see Bartus et al. 1982).

It is reasonable to conclude that the NGF-cholinergic, trophic-transmitter unit is central to contextual-spatial memory. NGF shapes and actively maintains the systems in which acetylcholine performs a mnemonic role. More generally, it is possible to move from trophic molecule to systems organization to mental module, memory, in a conceptually coherent fashion. The rules governing NGF synthesis and release, the kinetics of receptor binding, and the biochemical reactions of second messenger systems in responsive basal forebrain neurons, for example, comprise one set of principles underlying systems organization of the brain. Consequently specific trophic molecules, exemplified by NGF, contribute to the blueprint governing the organization of behavior and mental function. The septo-hippocampal-NGF-cholinergic hardware is not separate from the spatial memory software. Characteristics of contextual-spatial memory are expressions of the structure and function of the foregoing molecules, systems, and connections. Hardware and software are inseparable.

Septo-hippocampal NGF and acetylcholine are indirectly related as architect and operating signal in this system; moreover, a more direct relation may exist. NGF increases cholinergic function in receptive basal forebrain neurons. NGF increases CAT activity and acetylcholinesterase, and it also increases cholinergic neuron size under certain conditions. Consequently NGF may enhance the cholinergic transmission that constitutes ongoing memory function. Memory is the state of the biological unit, which consists of trophic, transmitter, and systems components that are indivisibly interdependent.

NGF and Other Brain Systems

While NGF specifically and selectively regulates the development and function of cholinergic populations in the basal forebrain-cortical system, mounting evidence suggests that the factor exerts actions on other brain systems as well. For example, cholinergic interneurons in the striatum respond to NGF with increased CAT activity in vivo and in vitro and express receptors (Martinez et al. 1985; Mobley et al. 1985). Moreover, the NGF and receptor genes are expressed in widely distributed brain areas, including olfactory bulb, cerebellum, and striatum, in addition to the forebrain-cortical system (Buck et al. 1987, 1988; Lu et al. 1989). Consequently the trophic factor may influence the ontogeny and function of multiple brain systems. At this early stage of investigation, the precise actions of NGF in these areas remain to be delineated, and behavioral consequences have yet to be defined. Nevertheless, it is already clear that NGF potentially affects multiple brain systems. Conversely, do multiple trophic factors govern function of brain systems?

Other Trophic Molecules in the Brain

NGF, the most fully characterized trophic factor, has been the focus of extensive study; emerging evidence also suggests that other factors govern survival and function of different neural systems. The list of potential factors is too long to permit complete enumeration in the context of this discussion. However, several examples are cited to indicate the rich possibilities for the regulation of systems development and function.

Recent studies indicate that fibroblast growth factor (FGF) supports the survival of striatal and cerebrocortical neurons in culture (Walicke et al. 1986; Walicke 1988; Walicke and Baird 1988; Morrison et al. 1986). The actions of this agent are pleiotropic, however, and angiogenesis and glial proliferation also appear to be induced. Specificity and selectivity, and potential interaction with other trophic and growth factors, remain to be elucidated. Similarly, epidermal growth factor (EGF) also exerts trophic actions on different central populations (Morrison et al. 1986), although normal physiologic roles remain to be defined. These two examples, among many others, indicate that molecules originally discovered and characterized elsewhere in the body also exert actions in the nervous system. It is reasonable to anticipate that a variety of defined peripheral signals will be found to regulate brain systems as well.

In addition to the discovery of "new" actions for old molecules, a number of "new" molecules have also been characterized in the nervous system. Ciliary neurotrophic factor (CNTF) was originally detected in ocular components and supported the survival of ciliary ganglion parasympathetic neurons that normally innervate the eye (Varon et al. 1979; Barbin et al. 1984; Manthorpe and Varon 1985). Molecular characterization revealed that CNTF is an acidic protein with a molecular mass of 22 kD, distinguishing it from NGF, EGF, and FGF (Manthorpe et al. 1986). The availability of pure preparations of the molecule is now allowing delineation of the spectrum of biologic effects. Recent work, for example, suggests that CNTF regulates mitosis and transmitter phenotype of sympathetic neurons, in addition to actions on ciliary neurons (Ernsberger et al. 1989). Consequently CNTF may simultaneously serve as a survival (trophic) factor, mitogen, and transmitter-regulating factor for different populations. The orthodox classification of factors by function appears to be dissolving.

Brain-derived neurotrophic factor (BDNF), originally purified from the pig brain, supports the survival of subpopulations of sympathetic and sensory neurons (Leibrock et al. 1989). Sequence analysis of the molecule indicates that it is a distinct entity, although it shares sequences with NGF. Future work will reveal whether NGF is but one of a family of trophic molecules. It is still unclear whether multiple gene families encode groups of trophic factors that regulate the development and function of brain systems.

It is abundantly clear, however, that the traditional distinction among trophic factors, growth factors, and transmitters is breaking down. A variety of molecules exert acute, millisecond-to-millisecond transmitter actions and also regulate long-term neuronal function. The classical transmitters, serotonin and acetylcholine, for example, also regulate nerve process (neurite) outgrowth and the survival of neuronal populations in culture. Insulin and the insulin family of growth factors that function as transmitters also regulate neurite outgrowth and the mitosis of neurons (DiCicco-Bloom and Black 1988). Calcitonin gene-related peptide (CGRP) serves as a transmitter and also regulates transmitter phenotypic expression (Mudge 1989; Denis-Donini 1989). The peptide transmitter vasoactive intestinal peptide (VIP) regulates neuronal mitosis, process outgrowth, and survival of sympathetic populations (Pincus et al. 1990).

These few examples, drawn from a rapidly expanding literature, suggest that traditional distinctions among transmission, growth, systems development, and function are ill framed. System use, with attendant transmission, may foster survival, growth, connectivity, and enhanced function in the future. Experience may alter function through the mediation of these molecular signals that govern transmission, growth, and trophism simultaneously. Environmental, epigenetic information may thereby influence the organization of systems and the behavior and mental states that are engendered. The quasi-permanent alteration of systems function by experience, with the consequent alteration of behavior and mental function, may be attributable to these trophic-transmitter-growth molecules. The dynamic relationship among environment, molecular signals, systems, and behavior may underlie aspects of learning and memory.

Chapter 8

Modularity of Brain Function: Psychologic, Anatomic, and Molecular Domains

Split-Brain Patients—Disconnection Syndromes—Disconnection and Modularity in Parkinson's Disease—Modularity in Subhuman Primates: Molar-Molecular Relationships—Learning without Mind—Psychologic Modules as Trophic Units?

Our discussion indicates that modularity of behavior—the organization of independent, component brain functions into coherent repertoires—is evident at the most fundamental neural level: organization of the genome. The sequential consideration of polyprotein organization and trophic factor-systems organization suggests that modularity is a feature of many levels of function of the nervous system. In fact, a number of levels that incorporate modularity are readily identifiable. Genomic modularity yields molecular modularity and compartmentalized biochemical and metabolic functions. Modular constitution of polyproteins, for example, leads to compound physiologic and behavioral states that consist of discrete components. In turn, systems organization of the brain comprises the substrate upon which the modular molecules act, resulting in modular behavior.

Modularity is evident at multiple phylogenetic, as well as functional, "levels." Modular organization is not restricted to the complex vertebrate nervous system but is also evident in the invertebrate. The egg-laying behavioral repertoire in the sea snail, indicates that both "simple" and "complex" systems exhibit modularity. Modular genes yield clusters of transmitter and trophic products that elicit behavioral modules at different levels of phylogenetic complexity.

How is modularity manifested at the most complex levels in the human and subhuman primate brain? Does modular function constitute an unbroken line of logic extending from the simplest to the most complex levels of neural organization? In fact, a number of the striking clinical syndromes described in the Introduction derive from modular organization of the human brain. Remarkable behavioral and mental dissociations are expressions of deranged modularity. We now analyze normal and abnormal function in humans to define the design of modularity in human cognition. We examine the contention that (apparently unitary) human brain states actually consist of component functions that are processed separately.

Initially we adopt a neural systems approach to examine modularity of human mentation and behavior. Data from split-brain patients are analyzed in terms of systems function and lateralization of brain function. These considerations lead naturally to a discussion of clinical disorders in which systems are separated—the so-called disconnection syndromes. The particular qualities of behavioral and mental decomposition in these disorders graphically illustrate the nature of normal modular integration. With this background, we discuss experimental studies in subhuman primates that focus on the systems basis of associative learning and memory. These observations are used to place modularity of higher cognitive function in a systems, transmitter, and trophic context. Our overall goal is to see how molecular interactions, in conjunction with systems organization, generate modularity of behavior and cognition.

Modularity in Split-Brain Patients

Observations based on many different clinical disorders and experimental paradigms support the contention that behavior and underlying brain function are organized in a modular fashion. The extensive work of Gazzaniga and colleagues with the well-known, split-brain patients has graphically demonstrated essential features of modularity in humans and its profound practical and theoretical consequences (for review, see Gazzaniga 1970, 1989; Gazzaniga and LeDoux 1978). For a number of decades, patients with debilitating epilepsy, in which seizure activity spreads from one hemisphere to the other, have been helped by a procedure that separates the two halves of the brain. Surgical transection of the connections between the hemispheres, the corpus callosum and anterior commissure, isolates each half-brain and prevents the spread of seizure activity (figure 8.1). Gazzaniga's ingenious studies take advantage of the fact that information from the left visual field goes only to the right hemisphere, while that from the right visual field is transmitted only to the left (figure 8.2). Surgical disconnection prevents the two hemispheres from communicating directly. Consequently neither hemisphere has access to visual cues presented to the other. The stage is set for asking some fascinating questions.

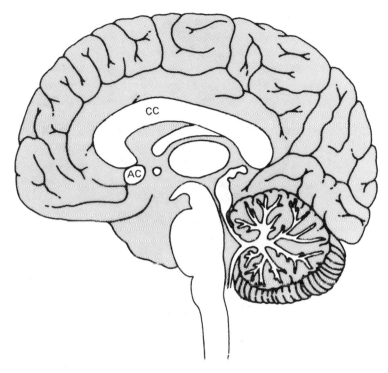

Figure 8.1
Sagittal view of the human brain, depicting the corpus callosum (CC) and the anterior commissure (AC). These are the fiber tracts that are transected in intractable epilepsy resulting in the so-called split brain. (After Gazzaniga 1970)

Flashing scenes or words to a single visual field can selectively stimulate the verbal left hemisphere or activate the mute right hemisphere. As expected, the left hemisphere easily reads messages and can report on them in exquisite detail. The right hemisphere, in contrast, can observe a scene and react but lacks the apparatus to report verbally. Moreover, surgical disconnection prevents the right brain from communicating directly with the left.

How does the whole patient act when information is flashed to each half-brain? In attempting to answer this question, Gazzaniga discovered a remarkable phenomenon. As expected, the verbal left brain accurately reported on words, messages, and scenes displayed to the right visual field. Information shown to the right brain only was handled differently. In a now-classic example, an extremely disturbing scene, showing a burning building with potential victims, was flashed to the right brain (left field). Although the mute brain was unable to

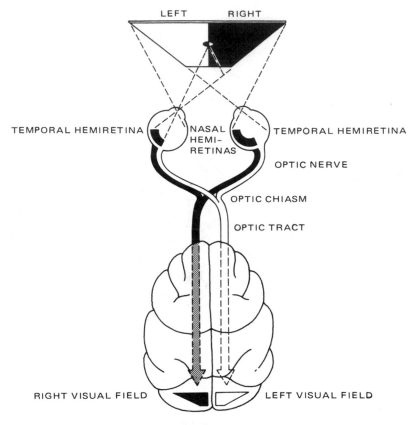

Figure 8.2
Visual information in split-brain patients. Note that information presented to each eye is projected almost equally to both hemispheres. Consequently visual information from the right visual field is projected only to the left hemisphere, and vice versa. (From Gazzaniga 1970)

describe the vision verbally, the patient became acutely agitated and anxious. When the patient was asked verbally what was wrong, a remarkable event occurred: the verbal left brain, not having observed the scene, made up a story. The patient (left brain) said that one of the scientists was making her uneasy and anxious. The left brain had concocted a theory to explain the cause of an internal state elicited by a scene shown only to the right brain. Trial after trial, control after control, and scene after scene, the same drama was enacted. The verbal left brain reproducibly fabricated explanations, theories, and hypotheses to explain actions and reactions originating in the inaccessible, mute, right brain.

Gradually a clear picture emerged. A psychologic function in the left brain is constantly attempting to make sense of a bewildering, largely inaccessible reality. Some agent in the dominant hemisphere does not tolerate the discontinuities, apparent paradoxes, and irregularities of existence and continually formulates, theorizes, and organizes events into a consistent, coherent, comprehensible reality (Gazzaniga 1970, 1985, 1989).

A variety of conclusions are warranted, but we shall focus exclusively on several immediately relevant to our context. First, the obvious asymmetry of the two hemispheres ipso facto argues for differential localization of different behavioral systems. Second, a specific psychologic module, which Gazzaniga terms the interpreter, is localized to the dominant hemisphere. Finally, the interpreter does not have access to right brain systems in the split-brain patients. Rather, the interpreter is a "superordinate" function that attempts to bring unity to a modular consciousness and to a discontinuous external reality. Normally the interpreter succeeds, and we experience a unified, integrated, mental life.

The far-reaching implications of these formulations are hardly restricted to "abnormal," split-brain patients. There is no reason to assume, out of hand, that disconnection is restricted to people who have undergone surgery. Rather, we are all disconnected to some degree. In all of us, multiple neural events and modules are inaccessible to language systems and the interpreter. Behaviors and mental states based on inaccessible variables are attributed to improper causes. Mood swings, for example, generated by hidden mechanisms, are frequently ascribed to incorrect antecedents. Gazzaniga has even suggested that phobias may be generated through interpretation of extreme emotional states, such as metabolically caused panic attacks. Storage of the intepretation in memory may result in phobic reactions long after the panic attacks have been medically controlled (Gazzaniga 1989). In summary, gross hemispheric separation has provided insight

into modular organization that shapes normal and abnormal mentation. We now examine the organization and relation of specific brain
subsystems that endow mental life with particular, and peculiar,
qualities.

Modularity and Disconnection Syndromes

In addition to disconnection of the two hemispheres, a variety of
neuropsychiatric syndromes result from disconnection of specific
modules resulting from human disease. Geschwind, in particular,
called attention to the central role of the brain area that receives
language input, termed Wernicke's area (figure 8.3; Geschwind 1965;
Galaburda et al. 1978). Functional separation of Wernicke's area from
other primary sensory areas of the brain results in a bizarre group of
disorders termed disconnection syndromes. One example may serve
to capture the flavor of these remarkable disorders.

One group of patients is unable to read (alexia) but can write per-
fectly well. They have alexia without agraphia, a syndrome affecting
the college professor described in the first paragraph of the Introduction. How can we understand the existence of such a counterintuitive
disorder? Patients with this problem have two brain lesions in combination that prevent visual information from reaching the receptive
speech area. Classically these individuals have a lesion in the left

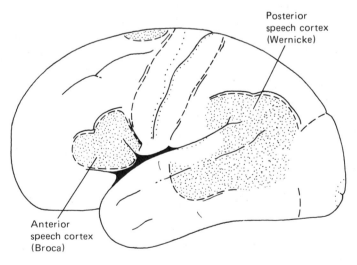

Figure 8.3
Language areas in the brain. (After Haymaker 1969)

occipital cortex, which receives visual information. They cannot see the right visual field and therefore cannot relay printed material from that field to the speech area. In addition, these patients have a lesion in the splenium (posterior portion) of the corpus callosum, which relays visual information from the left visual field to the speech area (figure 8.4). As a result, the receptive speech area is entirely cut off from visual information, leading to alexia. However, since execution of language function, such as speaking or writing, originates from a different region, the motor speech area (Broca's area), writing is not impaired. The syndrome of alexia without agraphia can be understood on the basis of fundamental, modular, neuroanatomical principles (for review, see Geschwind 1965).

Based on this brief description, we might predict that disconnection of Wernicke's area from other sensory modalities will lead to other unusual syndromes. The expectation is warranted. Pure word deafness—the inability to understand the spoken word, even though hearing, reading and writing are normal—results when Wernicke's area is separated from auditory input. Tactile aphasia, the inability to name an object simply by palpating it, results from the separation of Wernicke's area from somesthetic sensory input (Geschwind 1965).

In summary, the peculiar form of these receptive aphasic syndromes results from the peculiar organization of particular brain systems. Wernicke's receptive speech area is located in the inferior parietal lobule. This association area makes its appearance in primates at the junction of cortical areas for vision, audition, and somesthetic sensation. The lobule forms nonlimbic, intermodal associations, such as visual-tactile, a capability that appears uniquely in primates. In all other animals, associations are exclusively limbic-limbic and limbic-nonlimbic. For example, fear-aggression or sexual drive–motor activity typify more primitive associational pairings. Geschwind (1965) has suggested that the inferior parietal lobule is a prerequisite for the development of speech precisely because it forms nonlimbic associations. Simply stated, then, disconnection syndromes in humans result when Wernicke's area is separated from other primary sensory areas. Disconnection prevents language processing of sensory input.

While we have focused on sensory-speech disconnection and hemispheric disconnection, it is apparent that, in principle, modular organization sets the stage for diverse disconnection syndromes. For example, disconnection of Wernicke's area from motor centers leads to bizarre behavioral abnormalities, termed apraxias. On the other hand, agnosias, or disorders of naming, result from other types of disconnections. For example, some patients are able to sort, match, and recognize colors but cannot name them. In sum, the very nature

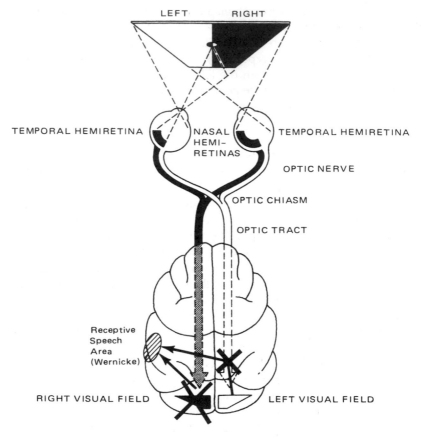

Figure 8.4
Anatomy of alexia without agraphia. Patients are unable to read since visual information from both hemispheres cannot gain access to the receptive speech area. However, patients are able to write since the motor language area is functional. Compare to figure 8.2. (After Gazzaniga 1970)

of symptom selectivity in disconnection syndromes has helped define the neuroanatomy of systems relations that result in modularity (for general discussion, see Geschwind 1965).

Although the importance of modularity in the generation of clinical disorders is obvious, implications for normal function are even more profound. The verbal systems of the brain, for example, normally have limited access to other brain systems. It is not surprising, consequently, that most individuals can provide only a vague account of internal emotional and physical states. Moreover, the interpreter stands ready to invent hypotheses and theories to explain inaccessible internal reality. Systems modularity plus interpreter action may be the formula that simultaneously leads the species to unprecedented creativity, confabulation, and self-delusion.

Proceeding from experimental animal models to modularity in humans, we have moved from a molecular to a systems approach. However, in rare, paradigmatic instances, the molecular and systems bases of modular derangement are apparent even in human disease. Brief reconsideration of Parkinson's disease may indicate how systems and transmitter organization yield modularity of motor function.

Disconnection and Modularity in Parkinson's Disease

Geschwind used the term disconnection to refer specifically to disor ders resulting from the separation of sensory areas from Wernicke's receptive speech area. Yet we have already described a "motor disconnection" syndrome in which the substantia nigra input to the striatum is interrupted: Parkinson's disease. This disorder has many of the general characteristics of conventional disconnection syndromes and therefore may be instructive (for an overview, see Fahn 1982). In Parkinson's, a constellation of motor symptoms exists in isolation, mimicking the apparently paradoxical nature of "true" disconnection syndromes. For example, Parkinson's results in rigid, bradykinetic, tremulous patients who are unable to initiate movement voluntarily. Paradoxically, these patients can effectively initiate complex, involuntary movements in emergencies, such as running out of burning homes, as mentioned in the introduction. Moreover, the Parkinsonian motor deficits are highly circumscribed, existing in the absence of paralysis, true weakness, or spasticity. Consequently, abnormalities in the execution of voluntary "motor programs" are unaccompanied by dysfunction of other motor modules. Deranged modularity results in strange motor dissociations, entirely analogous to the sensory-language dissociations Geschwind described.

Potential molecular bases of Wernicke's disconnection remain to be defined. However, in the case of Parkinson's, a number of underlying molecular mechanisms have been identified. First, nigrostriatal dopamine depletion is largely responsible for the signs and symptoms observed in this disorder. Moreover, multiple molecular abnormalities may result in dopamine dysfunction. Inhibition of dopamine synthesis, vesicular storage, release, or decreased number or affinity of dopamine receptors may result in the disconnection syndrome that we term Parkinson's disease. Moreover, different transmitters elicit antagonistic motor effects. For example, dopamine mediates hyperkinesia (increased movement) and improvement of the Parkinsonian symptoms. In contrast, cholinergic agents worsen the motor symptoms by precipitating hypokinesia (reduced and slowed movement). Different transmitter species differentially regulate the execution of a specific motor module. Indeed, normal function of this specific module depends on the precise balance of dopaminergic and cholinergic mechanisms. Dopamine in the nigrostriatal projection pathway ameliorates Parkinsonian deficits, whereas acetylcholine in striatal interneurons exacerbates the dysfunction. The general significance of this antagonistic transmitter relationship, however, extends far beyond any single disease.

The function of behavioral modules may now be described in terms of systems and molecules simultaneously. The reciprocally connected nigrostriatal system subserves one motor program module, and the role of two (of many) transmitters may be delineated with some precision. In this system, dopamine functions as a hyperkinetic agent. Increasing dopaminergic activity results in progressively increasing movement, ultimately resulting in the emergence of abnormal, extra (adventitious) movements characteristic of chorea, athetosis, and related disorders (see figure 4.4). Increased cholinergic function, in contrast, reduces movement, leading to immobility and frozen postures, in the extreme. The motor module is incorporated in the neural system, and its execution is governed by the balance of fully defined transmitter molecules. The neural systems and molecular signals basis of behavioral modularity can be defined in detail. Employing a similar strategy, we now consider learning and memory in subhuman primates to begin integrating the molecular and systems basis of modularity in cognitive function.

Modularity in Subhuman Primates: Some Molar-Molecular Relationships

In pioneering studies, Mishkin and coworkers are examining higher memory processing in subhuman primates (for review, see Mishkin

1982). Their work supports the existence of psychologic modularity in these species and is beginning to delineate critical transmitter functions. In summary, two distinct pathways that process visual information emerge from the occipital (visual) cortex (Mishkin et al. 1984). The ventral pathway projects to the temporal lobe and then to the limbic system and subserves pattern recognition (The "what" of an object; figure 8.5). The dorsal pathway, which projects to relays in the parietal and frontal lobes, is concerned with spatial discrimination (the "where" of an object; figure 8.5). Both the dorsal and ventral systems ultimately project to the amygdala and hippocampus, which together play a key role in the formation of visual memories (figure 8.5).

Combined amygdalectomy and hippocampectomy result in profound global amnesia for visual object recognition. In the relays from occipital cortex to temporal cortex to amygdala and hippocampus, sensory processing is thought to occur through orthograde activation, whereas memory processing occurs through retrograde activation (figure 8.6). That is, normal impulse activity traveling from occipital cortex to temporal lobe to limbic system and basal forebrain constitutes the forward-going sensory pathway. In contrast, retrograde impulses are

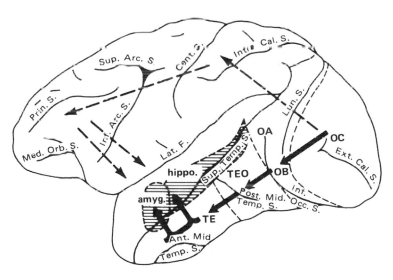

Figure 8.5
Processing of visual information in primates. Note that visual information in this depiction flows through two major pathways from the occipital cortex (OC). The ventral pathway is represented in detail with cortical areas OB, OA, and TEO and the most distal cortical temporal area, TE. From TE, information flows to the amygdala. (Adapted from Mishkin 1982)

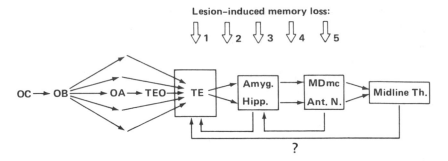

Figure 8.6
Schematic representation of orthograde and retrograde processes in visual information
flow and visual recognition memory. Visual information flows from primary visual area
OC through visual areas OB, OA, and TEO to TE in the temporal cortex. Information
is then relayed to the amygdala and hippocampus and subsequently to the thalamus,
consisting of MDmc, the magnocellular portion of the dorsomedial nucleus, and Ant.
N., the anterior nuclei. Finally, information is relayed to the midline thalamic nuclei.
Retrograde processes are represented by backward arrows and may represent activation
of memory. (From Mishkin 1982)

thought to activate the stored representations, which comprise
memory.

Other sensory modalities also feed into the amygdala and hippocampus. Somatosensory, auditory, gustatory, and tactile as well as
visual information are relayed to the amygdala and hippocampus. The
amygdala and hippocampus serve to associate this cross-modal information that is not on the immediate, conscious, sensory surface.
Amygdala and hippocampus thus free the organism from a world
bounded by immediate perception. These limbic structures emanci-
pate the individual from an eternal present and yield an associative,
historical being (Mishkin 1982; Mishkin et al. 1984).

These recognitive, associative processes constitute the basis of
thought, utilizing associated memories. The amygdala and hippocampus subserve representational, informational learning. And here we
encounter one of the most striking instances of dissociations resulting
from modular organization: combined destruction of the amygdala
and hippocampus, with total impairment of associational thought,
does not affect habit formation, classical conditioning, instrumental
conditioning, or procedural learning (such as bike riding). The individual "learns" stimulus-response bonds without a "mind." Mishkin
(1982; Mishkin et al. 1984) offers this instance of modularity as a
resolution of the apparently contradictory behaviorist and cognitivist
accounts of reality. Behaviorist processing involves the cortico-stria-

tum and cerebellum, as elegantly demonstrated by Thompson and colleagues (1986); cognitivist processes, of course, are amygdaloid and hippocampal. This is but one striking example of how the modular nature of mentality may give rise to seemingly inconsistent explanations of reality (for additional overview, see Squire 1986).

Modularity of mental function, and specifically the distinction between representational memory and stimulus-response bonds, extends from the systems to the molecular levels. Appreciation of molecular specificity requires additional description of the pathways involved.

The amygdala and hippocampus project to the large population of cholinergic neurons at the base of the forebrain, comprising the nucleus basalis magnocellularis, the medial septal nucleus, and the nucleus of the diagonal band of Broca (figure 8.6; see chapter 7). Lesions of these cholinergic neurons result in amnesia, as does treatment with scopolamine, a cholinergic antagonist (chapter 7). In contrast, cholinergic antagonists do not affect the formation of stimulus-response bonds. Consequently the transmitters subserving these two different types of memory are different.

We now expand our consideration of the role of the trophic-transmitter unit introduced in chapter 7. The basal forebrain cholinergic neurons clearly serve a variety of associational memories, in addition to the contextual-spatial memories described in the previous chapter. The potential roles of NGF and acetylcholine consequently include mediation of a spectrum of representational learning. Viewed in conjunction with the discussion in chapter 7, we tentatively conclude that NGF contributes to the formation and maintenance of a brain system that subserves representational, associational memory but not stimulus-response memory.

This functional module of neurons specifically and selectively expresses the panoply of molecules that confer NGF responsiveness; the module is also dependent on NGF for normal function. Modularity of function is associated not only with commonality of transmitter phenotype but also with a common requirement for a specific trophic molecule in this instance. Consequently, modularity has a molecular, trophic, and transmitter reality, as well as an anatomic systems reality. We are now in a position to relate trophic and transmitter function at the molecular level to systems integrity and mental function. Further, an understanding of these relationships permits tentative modeling of mental disease.

The basal forebrain neurons, through the actions of acetylcholine in the cerebral cortex, are necessary for the formation of associational memories. In turn, the integrity of this cholinergic system is dependent on NGF elaborated in the cortex. This associational memory module is distinguished by cholinergicity, responsiveness to NGF, apparent dependence on NGF, and cortical innervation.

These distinguishing characteristics have allowed speculation regarding potential pathogenetic mechanisms governing mental disease. This particular module is one of the most prominent cell groups that degenerates in Alzheimer's disease. Not surprisingly, memory deficits predominate early in this tragic, dementing illness. Based on the extensive evidence already discussed, it has been suggested that an abnormality of NGF synthesis, metabolism, reception, or signal transduction may contribute to the prominent degeneration of basal cholinergic neurons in this illness. The resultant cholinergic deficits would then contribute to the profound amnesia characteristic of Alzheimer's. While this formulation remains conjectural, it may have useful implications for new therapeutic approaches to Alzheimer's disease. Moreover, it may lead to a more general understanding of the bases of a variety of late-life, degenerative neurologic diseases.

NGF therapy may abort or reduce basal cholinergic degeneration, even if a primary deficiency of the factor is not causative. It certainly would be worthwhile to determine whether NGF treatment can prevent the destructive effects of excitotoxins, radiofrequency, and electrolytic lesions, all of which have been used to generate animal models of the disease. In other words, NGF administration may be beneficial whether or not it plays a primary pathogenetic role.

More generally, using NGF and Alzheimer's disease as a model, we may potentially approach an understanding of a variety of seemingly dissimilar late-life, degenerative neurologic diseases. For example, are motor neuron (Lou Gehrig's) disease, Pick's, Parkinson's, and olivo-pontocerebellar atrophy attributable to derangements in specific trophic interactions, including deficits of trophic factors? Conversely, do derangements in the same trophic interactions at different times in life result in seemingly separate and distinct disorders? In other words, does the same molecular defect, occurring at different stages of life, cause Werdnig-Hoffman's disease (infantile motor neuron death), a classical "developmental" disorder, and "degenerative" motor neuron disease? Although these questions are formidable, they are all approachable in experimental animals and through the use of human postmortem material.

Elucidation of the molecular basis of modularity may provide insights into clinical, as well as basic neurobiologic, mechanisms. Although information is rudimentary, rapid advances in this area hold the hope for far-reaching progress.

Conclusions

Our discussions indicate that modularity of behavior, a concept that arose from the study of humans and subhuman primates, has a physical reality in the brain. Modules may be defined anatomically, as in the cases of Wernicke's speech area and the basal forebrain nuclei. Moreover, in the latter, the module consists of neurons that use a common transmitter, acetylcholine. Finally, this anatomic-transmitter-behavioral module is selectively responsive to a specific trophic agent, NGF. Consequently modularity as a psychologic construct has a physical reality that serves to link molecular mechanisms, including NGF production, with cholinergic stimulation, systems function, and normal associative memory. Elucidation of underlying molecular mechanisms may indicate how modularity arises developmentally and phylogenetically and how functional integrity is maintained during maturity.

Chapter 9

Symbols and Regulatory Biology

Biological Function as Context—E. Coli Food Seeking—Tetrahymena and Euglena—Primitive Metazoan Effector Molecules—Slime Mold Communication—Parazoa (Sponges) and "Neural Function"—Behavior without Nervous Systems—Trophic Function in Hydra—Unity of Behavior and Metabolism

To approach brain function, we have focused on the existence of multiple levels in the hierarchy that constitutes brain and mind. A basic, underlying, interactive molecular level has been identified. The molecular level contains some of the basic units of higher neural function. In the normal nervous system, however, the multiplicity of levels and their multifarious interactions obscure many of the critical, elemental characteristics of molecular processes. To attain increased resolution through simplification, we turn to less complex organ systems and, in the limiting case, to single cells themselves. Conversely, we may ask whether effector molecules can be identified in unicellular organisms and whether these molecules serve a sensorimotor function even in such primitive forms. Insights may help place information-carrying molecules in the larger perspective of life itself and provide clues to the origins of neural function.

Neurotransmission is part of the larger process of information flow and the alteration of function in biologic systems. To survive, all cells presumably must be capable of information reception, processing, storage, and communication. These faculties are required for unicellular life as well as life of complex metazoa. Can we gain additional insights by attempting to place neural function in the broader context of biological regulation? More specifically, can we identify effector molecules and symbols in nonneural cells? By examining simple forms, the essential features of molecular transduction may be grasped, devoid of the confounding complexities of higher nervous systems. Our goal, then, is to determine whether regulatory molecules in simple cellular systems transduce environmental demands into altered metabolism and behavior and whether neural function is present even in the absence of conventional nervous systems.

In search of simplicity, we turn initially to an organism that has served succeeding generations of scientists well, the bacterium *E. coli*. Protein starvation of this unicell leads to increased intracellular concentrations of cAMP (regarded, incidentally, as a putative adenosinergic transmitter in higher forms), which stimulates flagellin synthesis, cell motility, and, hence, food-seeking behavior (figure 9.1; Yokota and Gots 1970). Even in a primitive prokaryote, a critical regulatory molecule that transduces information can be identified. Although bacteria do not possess a conventional nervous system, molecular regulatory symbols are already playing a role in the strategy of life.

Can we follow the cyclic nucleotide thread through a number of unicells in the hope of discerning a parallel or even a relationship to mind-brain molecules in higher organisms? Indeed, the photoheterotroph Euglena contains the molecular apparatus to process the phosphonucleotides; adenylate cyclase, cAMP, phosphodiesterase, and phosphokinase have all been identified (Keirns et al. 1973). It is of particular interest that although catecholamines are not detectable in this species, adenylate cyclase can be stimulated by exogenous catecholamines (Keirns et al. 1973). These and similar observations raise the intriguing possibility that molecules such as cAMP and related enzymes evolved as effectors in unicells and very early were sensitive to potential transmitters, the catecholamines. This contention is consistent with the observation that the protozoan *Tetrahymena pyriformis* exhibits adenylate cyclase activity and cAMP formation, which are stimulated by epinephrine and serotonin, amines endogenous to the organism (Rosensweig and Kindler 1972; Janakidevi et al. 1966). In *Tetrahymena*, the amino acid metabolites appear to regulate cellular growth and glucose metabolism (Blum 1970). Adenylate cyclase from *Phycomyces sporangiophore*, a giant, single-celled eukaryotic fungus, is

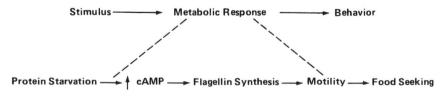

Figure 9.1
A metabolic-behavioral chain in *E. coli*.

stimulated by dopamine and epinephrine. cAMP appears to regulate the light-induced growth response in this organism (Cohen et al. 1980). Finally, adenylate cyclase has been detected in such varied unicells as *Brevibacterium liquifaciens*, *Saccharomyces fragilis*, *Neurospora crassa*, and *Acanthomeba palestensis* (Hirata and Hayaishi 1967; Sy and Richter 1972; Flawia and Torres 1972; Chlatkowski and Butcher 1973).

To summarize, these observations indicate that effector molecules, such as cAMP and adenylyl cyclase, play critical roles in the life of primitive forms, converting intracellular and environmental demands into altered behavior. Moreover, the enzyme appears to be sensitive to catecholamines even in primitive organisms that lack the amines. Although we are dealing with unicells that are highly evolved, we may speculate that phylogenetically, cyclase was potentially sensitive to catecholamines even before their evolutionary appearance. Relatively minor chemical changes in the naturally occurring amino acids tyrosine and tryptophan, yielding the catecholamines and indole amines, respectively, may have conferred selective advantages upon the cells in which they initially arose. Monoamines may have provided increased specificity and selectivity in the environmental regulation of cellular metabolism. Even in primitive monera and protista, sensorimotor molecules functioned as symbols (Tomkins 1975), defining sets of environmental or internal conditions and transducing this information into metabolic and behavioral processes. This abstract biochemical logic represents the essence of complex metabolic regulation and forms the basis for neural and endocrine function.

Metazoan Effector Molecules and Neural Function

As opposed to protistan progenitors, metazoa are faced with the problem of intercellular synchronization within a single organism, and this is accomplished through intercellular communication. Cell-to-cell signaling is largely achieved through the mediation of these same effector molecules and may be the forerunner of the conventional nervous system. A primitive stage in the elaboration of communication is represented by cellular interactions of the slime mold, *Dictyostelium*. In this species, starvation causes cAMP release by individual myxamoebas, which in turn promotes cellular aggregation, formation of a multicellular colony, and spore production (for review, see Devreotes 1989). In this instance, a critical intracellular regulator functions as an intercellular message. Moreover, association of unicells in colonies is hardly unique to slime mold; on the contrary, it is the rule in bacteria and may be partly mediated by intercellular signals, although most remain to be identified. The use of a normal intracellular message as an intercellular message is a particularly parsimonious and conservative biological strategy.

Intercellular communication in *Dictyostelium* is strikingly similar to that in advanced, true nervous systems. The intercellular signal. cAMP, elicits chemotaxis, morphogenesis, and selective gene expression by interacting with specific receptors on the cell membrane (Devreotes 1989). Moreover, the receptors are remarkably similar to the beta-adrenergic catecholamine receptor, exhibiting seven putative membrane-spanning domains and a serine- and threonine-rich COOH terminus. Similarly, the receptors are coupled to G proteins and to adenylyl cyclase, as are catecholaminergic receptors in the mammalian nervous system. The basic principles of signal-receptor organization, which characterize neural function, are present in the relatively simple *Dictyosteleum*.

To recap, in slime mold, as in prokaryotic unicells, intercellular molecular signals serve transducer functions. In the examples discussed, an environmental stimulus or condition elicits the elaboration and secretion of a specific signal that alters behavior of receptive cells. Shorn of layers of complexity and many levels of function, the rudiments of neural communication can be detected. Embedded in the fabric of some of the simplest forms of life, effector molecules regulate behavior. It certainly is of interest that cAMP, the prototypical, intracellular, neurohumoral second messenger, plays a prominent role in intercellular signaling in simple forms. There is a distinct possibility that effectors arose early in evolution, antedating the appearance of transmitter molecules proper, and constitute the progenitors of the conventional nervous system.

Complex Metazoan Forms

Metazoa may be classified according to several schemes (Whittaker 1969; Mayr 1981). To pursue our questions regarding the place of transducer molecules in very different life forms, modes of nutrition are particularly important. Photosynthetic plants, absorptive fungi, and ingestive animals comprise categories (Whittaker 1969; Mayr 1981) that are especially relevant to our interests. Ingestion in animals implies evolution of the motile, food-seeking life, which in turn may have contributed to the selection of sensorimotor mechanisms capable of perceiving and responding to food. Ingestive life placed a premium on rapidity of intercellular synchronization and communication and may have been a key determinant leading to the emergence of conventional neural mechanisms. Conversely, in plants and fungi, using principally photosynthetic and absorptive nutritional strategies, the value of neural mechanisms may have been limited.

Within the set of regulatory molecules, a subset with particular properties is advantageous for use in neural communication. Effector molecules that elicit **rapid** effects and that are metabolically **labile** are critical. While it is apparent that rapidity of effects is a sine qua non for certain aspects of neural communication, the importance of lability may be less evident. However, metabolic lability ensures that signals are evanescent, allowing vast amounts of information transfer over brief periods of time. Simultaneously, however, lability places constraints and demands on the nervous system. For example, lability limits the distances over which neurons can communicate with receptive cells, favoring point-to-point interactions. As individual animals increase in size phylogenetically, elaboration of long cellular processes in the form of axons represents one solution to the problem of proximate interactions. Extension of this logic leads to a system of unprecedented complexity in which intercellular connections assume critical importance in the generation of specificity of communication.

Lability and rapidity of action are not simply intrinsic properties of the transmitter molecules themselves but, in addition, depend on cellular mechanisms that ensure rapid delivery, response, and inactivation. Accordingly, mechanisms of biosynthesis, storage, delivery, inactivation, and response are central to neural function. In turn, each of these loci is a potential site for regulation by effector molecules. This formulation also represents a blueprint for the organization of neurotransmitter mechanisms. Can we trace the emergence of the nervous system in metazoa to assess the plausibility of these contentions?

A Parazoan Nervous System?

If true transmitters arose in primitive monera and protozoa, prior to the emergence of neurons, transmitter molecules and mechanisms should be detectable in the most primitive metazoa, whether or not neurons are present. The porifera (sponges) are the most primitive extant phylum of multicellular organisms and are not even eumetazoan ancestors. These parazoa do not exhibit stable histochemical differentiation but rather consist of a loose association of ectomesenchymal cells (De Ceccatty 1974). It is generally maintained that sponges do not contain neurons or neural mechanisms (Lentz 1966). Rather, as described in the classic work of Parker (1919), sponges contain epithelio-muscular cells at the pore and oscular sphincters, which, by contracting, regulate water flow through the channels of the organism.

Parker suggested that such effector cells preceded appearance of neurons and the nervous system. Subsequent authorities have subscribed to the view that sponges are indeed preneural (De Ceccatty 1974).

Are sponges truly "preneural," or is a simple nervous system already emerging in this, the most primitive extant metazoan? We focus on two particularly interesting cells: the spindle-shaped mesenchymal cells, which are adjacent to the pinacocytes and choanocytes (Hisada 1957; Franquinet and Martelly 1981), and large multipolar cells, which are abundant in the collar below the osculum (Lentz 1966, 1968, pp. 52–68). Both cells contain a number of potential transmitter molecules, including norepinephrine, epinephrine, serotonin, and "neurosecretory substance" (figure 9.2; Lentz 1966, 1968). Moreover, acetylcholinesterase and monoamine oxidase, transmitter-metabolizing enzymes, have been detected in these two cell types. Consequently, transmitter processing may occur. Finally, both cell types have small granular vesicles, measuring 1000–1700 Å, that may store putative transmitter (Lentz 1966). Consequently, cells in the allegedly "preneural" sponge contain transmitter molecules, appropriate metabolic enzymes, and specialized storage vesicles.

Of equal interest is the presence of **specialized intercellular junctions** between cells within the mesenchyme. The simplest involves junctions of parallel cell membranes with a separation of 100–150 Å. In some instances dense granules are observed adjacent to the membrane in one of the cells, with cell separation of 100–125 Å (Lentz 1968, pp. 34–45). In other specialized junctions, electron-dense material is interposed between the cell membranes (Lentz 1968, pp. 34–35). These junctions bear striking resemblance to primitive synapses.

In summary, intracellular neurohumours, storage vesicles, and specialized intercellular junctions, exhibiting some of the features of synapses, are present in the "preneural" sponge. These observations suggest that porifera represent a transitional, not "preneural," stage, in which neural traits and mechanisms for intercellular communication are emerging. Thus, even in the most primitive existent metazoan, neural characters are detected. Further, in sponges the conventional small molecule transmitters, such as norepinephrine, appear to be localized to the same cells as "neurosecretory substance" (Lentz 1968, pp. 52–68). Consequently, multiple putative transmitters may have coexisted in cells even before the advent of the definitive nervous and endocrine systems.

To summarize, sponges appear to be a transitional form in which molecular and subcellular structural elements of the nervous system are beginning to emerge. However, the porifera, the most primitive extant metazoan, lack conventional nervous systems at the macrocel-

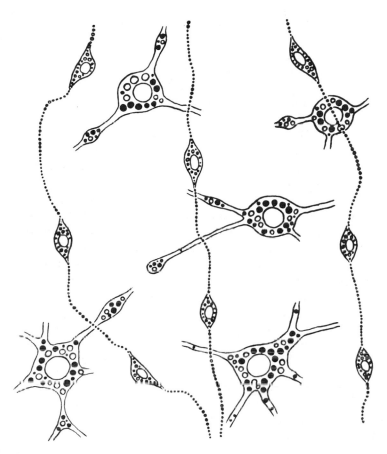

Figure 9.2
Transmitter storage vesicles in sponge cells. The vesicles, represented by spheres within the cells, have been revealed by epinephrine and norepinephrine staining. Two cell types stain positively and are represented as the large multipolar cells and the small bipolar cells. (From Lentz 1968)

lular level. This represents a unique opportunity to examine the function and relationship of the most basic units of neural mechanisms in the absence of the confounding complexity of levels that constitute the nervous system itself. A variety of experimental approaches may yield remarkable insights concerning the function of basic neural units. What is the extent and character of physiologic interactions among different cell types in sponges? How do these interactions affect behavior in sponges? This primitive metazoan is ideal for evaluating relationships among specific transmitters, receptors, and well-defined behaviors. The availability of numerous receptor agonists and antagonists makes this a realistic goal.

What is the relationship between the most basic molecular and cellular units of neural function and behavior, in the absence of the nervous system itself? Does behavior, paradoxically, antedate the phylogenetic appearance of the conventional nervous system? Are we simply stretching the definition of behavior to the point of triviality? In fact, this does not seem to be the case. Even in the instance of the simple repertoire exhibited by *E. coli*, it is apparent that the induction of motility and food seeking by cAMP constitutes behavior. Here, in this simple prokaryote, we gain a view of the crux: **at the most elemental level, behavior and metabolism are indistinguishable.** There is no simple, crisp divide between these two fundamental processes of life. Within the regulatory biology that is cellular metabolism, the rudiments of behavior are evident. At this basic level, categorical distinctions between metabolism and behavior are meaningless. In the sequence from protein starvation to elevation of cellular cAMP to increased flagellin synthesis to induced motility and food seeking, metabolism and behavior merge (figure 9.1).

There is no reason to assume that the absence of easy categorical distinctions is restricted to primitive forms. Rather, it is simply easier to detect unity in these relatively well-defined organisms. At the very least, we should approach the higher metazoan nervous system with caution. No a priori categorical distinctions should be accepted in the far more complex higher nervous system regarding behavior and cellular (neural) metabolism.

Coelenterates and the Conventional Nervous System

Coelenterates are the most primitive phylum in which a conventional nervous system is definable. In the coelenterate hydra, the nerve "net" appears to influence function of nematocysts, which impale and entwine prey prior to digestion. Feeding represents the most complex behavior of this coelenterate and is largely under neural control. Mechanical stimulation appears to cause nematocyst discharge through neurochemical mediation (Lentz 1968, pp. 44–45), and the transmitters acetylcholine, epinephrine, norepinephrine, serotonin, and histamine cause discharge in the presence of mechanical stimulation. The nematocysts are also capable of independent effector action, since the nervous system is not required for discharge. In other words, the primitive nervous system appears to enhance the actions of effectors already present, thereby increasing synchronization with the organism as a whole.

The general outlines of a biological scheme are beginning to take form. In bacteria, effector molecules, such as those of the adenylyl cyclase system, are detectable in the absence of neurotransmitters. Yet even in *E. coli,* the cAMP effector transduces the biologic state, starvation, into altered behavior—increased motility and food-seeking actions. In Euglena, cyclase is sensitive to exogenous catecholamines, although endogenous amines are not detectable. Finally, in the protozoan Tetrahymena, the effector cyclase system is regulated by epinephrine and serotonin, which are present in the organism. In unicells of increasing complexity, effector molecules initially appear and regulate behavior independently, subject only to external or internal conditions. With increasing complexity, transmitter molecules make their appearance and regulate the preexisting effectors, adding precision and synchronization of different metabolic functions. A parallel scheme is discernible in multicellular organisms of increasing complexity. In hydra, for example, the effector nematocysts can function independently or under the control of transmitters. Neurochemical regulation adds precision and synchrony. In general terms, effectors appear initially and serve a transducer function. With increasing complexity the effectors fall under the regulation of transmitters and the nervous system, conferring increased precision, specificity, and synchrony. Thus far we have focused on rapid communication in primitive organisms with or without simple nervous systems. However, it is now well recognized that the nervous system also subserves long-term communication and regulation in the form of growth and trophic effects. Can we identify growth and trophic interactions in primitive nervous systems and define the molecular messages involved?

Primitive Systems: Growth and Trophic Function

In addition to the role that neurons play in feeding behavior in hydra, the nervous system also governs histogenetic pattern formation and regeneration. Early work indicated that neurosecretory granules discharge during regeneration and appear to regulate growth and differentiation during the process of regeneration (Lentz and Bennet 1963; Lentz 1965a, 1965b; Lesh and Burnett 1966). Isolated granules, obtained by differential centrifugation, cause the development of supernumerary heads in excised midsegments of hydra, and the chemical factor that induces head formation is trypsin sensitive and dialyzable. Recently the head activator itself has been isolated and fully characterized (Schaller 1983). The molecule is an eleven amino acid polypeptide with the sequence

pGlu-Pro-Pro-Gly-Gly-Ser-Lys-Val-Ile-Leu-Phe.

Interestingly, a polypeptide of the identical sequence has been isolated from bovine and human hypothalami, raising the possibility that this ancient neuropeptide plays a role in the brain of higher organisms.

Calculations based on degree of purity and molecular weight indicate that the head activator in hydra is extremely potent, exerting physiological effects at 10^{-13} M. What are these physiological effects at the cellular level? The molecule has at least two specific effects: it stimulates cells to divide in a head-specific manner, and it influences cells to differentiate into components of the head itself. More specifically, during the S-phase of the cell cycle, the activator channels interstitial stem cells to differentiate along the nerve cell line. Since nerve cells themselves elaborate the head activator, the molecule functions in an autocatalytic manner, eliciting the formation of head nerve cells that, in turn, elaborate additional head activator.

Neurotrophic and growth regulation of head morphogenesis is more complex and precise than indicated by considering head activator alone. Nerves also secrete an inhibitor of head activation, and it is the ratio of activator to inhibitor that determines whether the cellular events that lead to head formation will transpire. The inhibitor appears to be a small molecule with a molecular weight of approximately 500 daltons. To summarize, highly specific growth regulation is performed by the nervous system in hydra, paralleling that observed in higher forms. In fact, head activation in hydra is mimicked by foot activation, in which the neural elaboration of a foot activator and an inhibitor determine whether foot morphogenesis occurs.

Among primitive nervous systems, growth regulation and trophism in hydra do not represent anomalies. For example, in planaria (worms), serotonin and dopamine stimulate regeneration from sectioned body segments through the mediation of increased adenylyl cyclase activity and altered DNA and RNA synthesis (Franquinet and Martelly 1981). This example also illustrates that growth and trophic regulation are not exclusively associated with neuropeptides but may be elicited by conventional small molecule transmitters. (Note that the cyclase system that we followed earlier in the chapter to monitor the emergence of the units of neural function also subserves neurotrophic function.)

In the most primitive extant conventional nervous systems, rapid electrogenic conduction and growth and trophic regulation are already detectable. Indeed, the two neural functions appear to have emerged together. Although far more work has been devoted to the elucidation of rapid communication, these observations suggest that trophic regulation may be as fundamental to the role of the nervous system as conduction of impulse activity. In fact, the presence of rapid communication and trophism in simple systems may indicate that the trophic modular unit is a feature of neural organization from the first. If this conjecture is valid, it may be possible to study the principles of modularity in very simple systems, eliminating many of the confounding variables and levels encountered in complex, higher nervous systems. It would be of extreme interest to trace the evolution of modularity itself to help define organizational foundations of the brain in complex forms.

Some Implications

It is apparent from this brief survey of simple systems that a number of seemingly obvious distinctions between structure and function are artificial. Further, concepts of discrete levels are misleading. Examination of relatively noncomplex animals indicates that biology and behavior are one. Simple forms of life, lacking the distracting complexity of higher forms, reveal that metabolism and behavior are fundamentally different aspects of the same process. For example, in the chain of events from protein starvation to increased cAMP to elevated flagellin synthesis to motility in E. coli, crude distinctions collapse (figure 9.1). Where does metabolism end and behavior begin? As we appreciate from our study of molecular processes, each of the events that has been identified in E. coli consists of multiple subevents. That is, the increase in cAMP is due to complex chemical reactions including adenylyl cyclase, ATP, phosphodiesterase, and others. The behavior, motility, consists of flagellar beating, which in turn is composed of multiple reactions in each flagellum, coordination among flagellae, and so forth, ultimately dependent on flagellin synthesis and the rise in cAMP.

In the most general terms, we may agree that protein starvation constitutes a stimulus to which motility is the response. However, beyond this uninformative simplification, categories tend to merge. Does motility begin with the increase in cAMP, the increase in flagellin synthesis, or the multiple processes involved in synchronized flagellar beating? Motility is the change of position in space resulting from all of these molecular interactions. More accurately, motility is the summation of a series of movements of molecules in space. Motility, the behavior that occurs in the microscopic domain, is simply a manifestation of molecular movements occurring in the submicroscopic domain. In this simple organism, the layers involved in the behavioral hierarchy collapse to form a series of chemical interactions. These processes may be regarded as metabolic reactions or may be "chunked" to comprise behavior. Nevertheless, even in this simple paradigm, we can define input stimuli, output behavioral responses, and intervening, causally related pathways. Perhaps the greatest complexity enters at the level of scientific description, not at the level of biological behavior. While the scientific endeavor may be organized into levels of investigation for methodological reasons, the research strategy should not be confused with the biological strategy. A chemical reaction or a molecule is literally simultaneously part of a metabolic pathway, part of a chemical response, and part of a behavior. It is not terribly informative to insist that it is more of a metabolic pathway than a behavior.

Our approach to behavior in E. coli requires a new description recognizing that a functional unit participates in multiple response domains simultaneously. The biological context, comprising the specific stimulus set and organism state, determines the response domains of which any single unit is a part. In the case of E. coli, the stimulus set, protein starvation, elicits increased cAMP and flagellin synthesis, which participate in the metabolic and behavioral motility response domains simultaneously. A symbol, such as cAMP, may move to different subsets of response domains at different times depending on the biological context. For example, cAMP may be restricted to a metabolic pathway when participating in phosphorylation of enzymes involved in intermediary metabolism. This model conforms to the provisional formulation outlined in chapter 1.

Chapter 10
Symbols, Self, and Subjectivity

Hierarchical Systems—Psychological Function Changes Molecules, Which Changes Psychological Function—Reciprocity and Multiple Levels—The Self in Space, the Self in Time, and the Social Self—Frontal Lobes and Reciprocal Connections—Schizophrenia and Derangement of the Self—Social Interaction

To trace neural function from molecules to behavior, we have implicitly employed a traditional, hierarchical model, identifying "levels." This construct has allowed tentative description of psychologic and behavioral modules in transmitter and trophic terms. The levels model has facilitated detection of a potential physical basis for the psychologic concept of modularity. However, have we really gained any insight into such elusive states as conscious awareness? What have our formulations contributed to an understanding of the sense of self? Is there, in fact, a deeper relationship among levels, symbols, and meaning that infuses self and subjectivity with a physical reality? In fact, the most critical properties of the nervous system remain to be described. And it is this explicit description that elucidates higher levels of mental function. The framework of this description directly concerns the nature of hierarchy in the nervous system and the relationship of functional levels. That the nervous system is organized hierarchically can scarcely be doubted. The ordering of function from genes to molecules, synapses, neurons, neuronal populations, neural systems, brains, organisms, groups, demes, and species is a theme that pervades our discussions. Modularity itself is a statement of hierarchic organization of brain function. However, it must be clear that the hierarchic structure of central interest is that of **control,** not simply **classification** (Grene 1987). The nervous system comprises elementary units contained in more complex units, such that elementary, low-level units constitute building blocks for structures at the complex, higher levels, and the higher levels constrain and control function at lower levels. Representation and meaning exist at multiple levels. Perhaps more important, information flows horizontally and vertically and may jump many levels at a time, either up or down. For example, high-level behavior alters the low-level molecules upon which the behavior is based. We illustrate these relationships in detail, since "jumping" of information across multiple levels endows mentality with some of its more elusive qualities. To begin understanding such complex mental structures as self and subjectivity, we consider how molecules that convey information underlie behavior and mental function and, conversely, how behavior and mental function change events on the molecular level.

It is the very fact that higher function, including behavior, mental state, and ideas, changes the molecular phenomena upon which higher function is based that, in the end, gives rise to the seemingly inexplicable qualities termed mind.

Having developed some familiarity with the vocabulary, experimental approaches, and concepts employed on the different levels of the mind-brain system, we now proceed with our inquiry in detail. Our objective is to begin with higher levels of function and determine whether phenomena at these levels alter succeedingly lower levels upon which the cognitive capacities are based. To revert to the computer metaphor, does high-level software actually change the lower-level hardware? If this does occur, should we begin thinking of the mind-brain cycle or sphere, as opposed to hierarchy (for an overview of hierarchy in biology, see Welch 1987)?

Psychologic Function

We have already been introduced to the interpreter, the psychologic module that organizes reality and elaborates theories to order internal and environmental stimuli. The interpreter does not tolerate ambiguity, discontinuity, or chance. Rather, this (superordinate) module constantly invents hypotheses to account for the ceaseless barrage of internal and external information. As we have seen, a faulty theory is far preferred to no theory at all. The line, if any, between insightful invention and fabrication does not seem to exist for the interpreter. So, on being presented with a frightening scene subliminally, the interpreter makes up a story to account for the attendant hypervigilance and anxiety experienced but not apprehended. Do hypervigilance and anxiety, and the elicited interpretation, alter the molecular processes upon which they are based?

The question brings us face to face with an extraordinary paradox. We have already discussed the role of the locus coeruleus in contributing to the attention-arousal-anxiety complex. The central role of the enzyme, tyrosine hydroxylase (TH), in locus function has been described. We have noted that environmental or internal "stress" increases locus discharge, resulting in biochemical induction of the rate-limiting enzyme. In turn, induction of the enzyme leads to enhanced synthesis of the amine transmitter and increased availability for release. But, in turn, increased locus activity and release lead to increased attention, vigilance, and anxiety at the psychological "level." Increased anxiety (including arousal and hypervigilance) may be perceived as threat by the interpreter, leading to enhanced locus activity and induction of TH, which leads to hypervigilance.

We have identified the physical basis in the mind-brain system of the "strange loops" postulated by Hofstadter in his metaphorical *Godel, Escher, Bach* (1979). The simplest depiction of this strange loop or continuous cycle is represented in figure 10.1. Locus activation begets arousal, attention, vigilance, potentially anxiety, and TH induction,

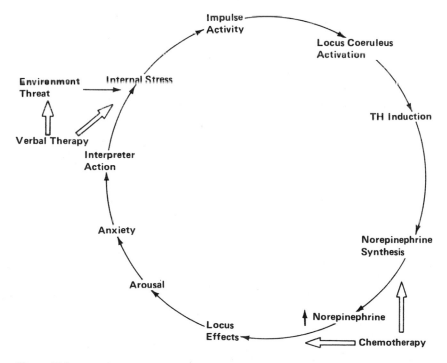

Figure 10.1
Brain function and molecular-behavioral-molecular loops. Schematic representation of information flow from environment to internal state, systems function, molecular regulation and behavior.

which begets interpretation as stress, which increases locus activity, and so forth. Psychological state reaches down to the very molecular level upon which the psychological state is based and changes that molecular substrate. The "levels," so easily defined verbally, are not separate and distinct in reality. Information flows from mental state to molecule and back. The psychological symbols hypervigilance and anxiety, and their cognitive interpretative symbols change the molecular symbol, TH, necessary for the genesis of the psychological symbol, anxiety.

Where does anxiety, the psychological experience, end and enzyme induction, the molecular reality, begin? In fact, our previous discussions have defined a number of the intermediate mechanisms driving this continuous cycle or strange loop. Cycles within cycles, symbols within symbols, and codes within codes are hidden in these mechanisms. It may be useful to reidentify these discrete mechanisms to help follow information flow among levels.

A Profusion of Levels

We review the molecular mechanisms involved in TH induction to define explicitly how high-level hypervigilance and anxiety may change the hardware on which they are based. Since all of the mechanisms have not yet been worked out in the locus, we borrow information derived from the study of the sympathoadrenal system. To recap, available evidence suggests that molecular regulation is similar in all of these catecholaminergic cell types. Insights obtained from the study of one of these cells may be applied to the others with a fair degree of certainty.

In summary, electrical discharge of the locus, which appears to be one cause of hypervigilance and anxiety, also induces TH, leading to the potential for increased anxiety. In catecholaminergic cells, impulse activity induces TH by increasing the level of messenger RNA coding for the TH enzyme. How many different levels are involved in this process? Although answers remain tentative, we are gaining an ever-clearer picture.

Impulse activity appears to accelerate the rate at which the TH messenger RNA is produced by other enzymes from the genomic DNA. A brief description of well-known DNA may help identify the levels involved in this mind-brain system and the location of symbolic function at different levels. DNA, of course, is a long string of connected molecules that comprises the code for the ultimate production of proteins, some of them enzymes (figure 10.2). Four specific molecules or "bases" make up the code: guanosine (G), cytosine (C), ad-

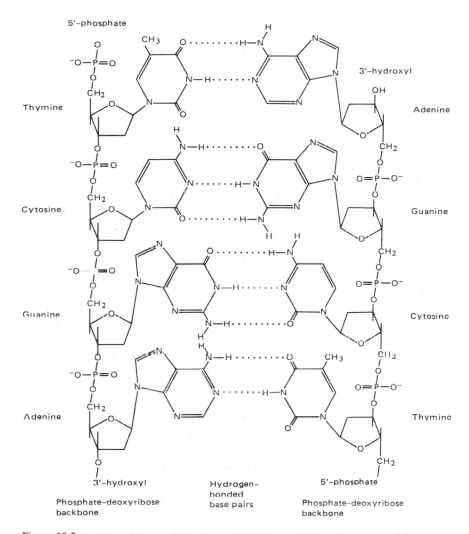

Figure 10.2
DNA symbols. Schematic representation of a small portion of the DNA double helix, depicting the matching base pairs, thymine, cytosine, guanine, and adenine, which are associated through hydrogen bonding. (From Lewin 1983)

enine (A), and thymidine (T). The coded information that leads to the synthesis of an enzyme protein such as TH is contained in the order of bases in the DNA molecule. In other words, DNA itself is another series of symbols at a fundamental level in the cell. How is TH synthesized from the DNA symbols?

Each series of three bases, or "triplet," encodes one amino acid unit in the final protein—in this case, TH. However, the DNA does not "translate" directly into protein but rather "transcribes" to an intermediate level, messenger RNA. The message is composed of different bases that pair in a complementary fashion with those of the DNA. After synthesis is complete, the message symbol is transported out of the nucleus of the cell into the cytoplasm where it is read, or translated, into the TH protein, or into a precursor protein, as in the case of the polyproteins. The molecular levels—their symbolic meaning and their interaction—do not end here.

Translation of the message into the protein occurs on the cytoplasmic ribosomes, is mediated by a series of cytoplasmic enzymes, and results in the attachment of individual amino acids in a linear string. The string of amino acids, known as the primary structure of the protein, in turn, contains additional information. The primary structure incorporates all the information necessary to dictate how the protein will fold up in three-dimensional space. And it is the three-dimensional conformation of the protein, its tertiary structure, that dictates biologic activity of the molecule. In the case of TH, the folding process produces an active catalytic site that binds the substrate, tyrosine, and hydroxylates it to form L-DOPA. Moreover, the folded TH contains additional sites that may be phosphorylated, changing the tertiary structure of the molecule, with consequent increases in the rate of the enzymatic conversion of tyrosine to L-DOPA.

Since TH is the rate-limiting enzyme in the synthesis of catecholamines, induction results in increased elaboration of transmitter and, in the case of the locus, enhanced target stimulation, and, presumably, increased arousal, hypervigilance, and anxiety. But anxiety initiated the complex of molecular events; anxiety increases locus discharge, which results in elevated transcription of message from DNA, leading to increased translation of message into protein amino acid sequence, which results in the three-dimensional folding of TH, increased transmitter synthesis, and further anxiety (figure 10.1).

Some Implications

Clearly this is an example in which high-level software symbols of a mental state change the low-level hardware symbols upon which the mental state is based. Biology becomes behavior, and behavior becomes biology. Indeed, biology is behavior, and behavior is biology. Environmental or internal exigencies drive the locus and are translated into biologic reality. Thoughts or environmental situations provoking anxiety are immediately translated into neural language. Environmental stimulus, mental state, behavior, and molecular mechanism are in constant interplay, forming an unbroken, continuous cycle (figure 10.1).

We can now begin to understand the artificiality of arbitrary distinctions between external environment and internal environment, mind and brain, and between such disciplines as psychiatry and neurology. Is it possible to change the biology of the brain by simply talking to an individual? Of course. To the extent that talk alters mental imagery that evokes attention, hypervigilance, and anxiety, thereby changing brain mechanisms, the biology of the brain will be altered precisely in the manner described in detail. Moreover, the interpreter stands ready to render its hypothesis, leading to additional potential changes in low-level, molecular hardware.

Let me be quite clear. In principle, verbal therapy, whether psychotherapy or in-depth psychoanalysis, has the capacity, as does drug therapy, to change the biology of the brain. The distinction is that each mode of therapy intervenes at a different point in the mind-brain cycle (figure 10.1). Both therapeutic modes change biology if they are to be efficacious. Verbal therapy owes its effectiveness to the fact that manipulation of the high-level software is capable of altering the low-level hardware of the brain. Further, the increasing use of combined verbal and drug therapy in psychiatry attests to the fact that intervention at several loci in the mind-brain cycle simultaneously is a successful strategy.

In addition to the therapeutic implications of this model, it also points to a number of conceptual difficulties that arise when contemplating such ideas as mind, self, and subjectivity.

Self and Subjectivity

With this background, we can begin to approach some of the high levels of function armed with a number of salient questions. What is the evidence, if any, that higher levels, such as the self, actually have a physical reality in the brain? What are the attributes of this putative entity on the high level that I am describing? Is there any method to tentatively localize aspects or components of the (? modular) self to areas or systems within the brain?

We all presumably have an apparently intuitive, subjective awareness of ourselves as discrete existences, separate and distinct from the
"outside." Of what does this special awareness consist? Instead of
launching into philosophical constructs, let us examine the evidence
from the pragmatic neurological clinic. Careful observation of patients
with neurological disorders over the past century has led to a relevant
storehouse of clinical-pathological correlation. Examination of this rec-
ord may help to characterize the attributes of a sense of self and yield
clues as to the underlying physical substrate ("lower level"), if any.

One important caveat is warranted: neurologic disorders are only
those dysfunctions that are so gross as to allow detection by our crude
methods. By employing the simplifying strategy of the neurological
approach, we will, perforce, sacrifice much of the subtlety and richness
that make up the self. Conversely, however, we hope to exclude
anecdote, bias, and armchair speculation.

A tentative, somewhat vague hypothesis may direct our attention
to the most significant spheres: the self is that collection of faculties
that allows recognition of the subjective entity, its distinction from
"not me," its continuity over time, its existence in space, and its ability
to act appropriately in the social (human) context.

What well-documented abnormalities shed light on the nature of
self at its high level and on the underlying physical substratum? A
constellation of relevant clinical abnormalities has been described.
Damage to the nondominant (usually right) parietal lobe leads to
several disturbances that reveal much about the characteristics of the
self (figure 10.3). Extensive lesions lead to neglect of the left half of
space, including the left half of the body. A patient shown his or her
own left arm or leg, for example, denies that it is part of him or her.
Some function in the nondominant parietal lobe apparently recognizes
left self and not self, makes the distinction, and is therefore critical for
a sense of physical integrity of the self. The parietal-self connection
does not end here (for an introductory overview, see Haymaker 1969).

These same patients also suffer from anosagnosia (Haymaker 1969);
they do not recognize that their selves are suffering from a disease.
Picture such a patient with left-sided paralysis or weakness and left-
sided sensory deficits, denying that he or she has any impairment.
Lying in a hospital bed, unable to move normally, surrounded by
doctors and nurses, the patient denies all abnormalities. It must be
stressed that these patients are not suffering from generalized cognitive abnormalities such as dementia. Clearly this represents a specific,
severe impairment of the sense of self.

To summarize, a faculty in the nondominant parietal lobe is necessary for the recognition of that part of the physical self in the opposite

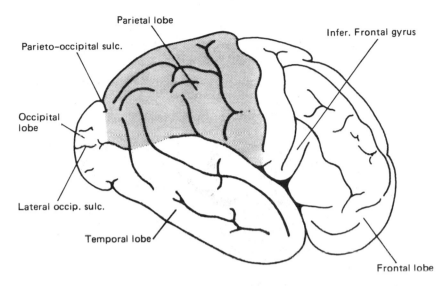

Figure 10.3
The nondominant parietal lobe. Diagram of the lobes on lateral surface of the cerebral hemisphere. (Adapted from Truex 1959)

side of space and is necessary for the recognition of abnormalities of the self. The principle is far more important than this particularity, however. **Components of the self and subjective awareness are localized to specific regions of the brain.** Although the precise neural subsystems have yet to be defined, a physical substratum for the most subjective of psychologic entities has been identified. It is reasonable to expect that ongoing investigation will define the levels, from neural system to transmitter molecules, that are associated with these functions of self in the nondominant parietal lobe.

Lesions in other areas of the brain derange other functions of the self. Frontal lobe dysfunction profoundly impairs the self in a social context (figures 10.4 and 10.5; Haymaker 1969; Adams 1962). A patient with frontal disease frequently loses the social graces that characterize the self in society. He or she has a flat affect, fails to greet a friend or newly introduced stranger appropriately, converses in an emotionless, colorless fashion, and loses the ability to bid farewell in socially accepted ways. Some of these patients suffer from the so-called frontal lobe bladder syndrome, urinating in public with an apparent total indifference to the impropriety of the act. This latter syndrome has been localized to bilateral paracentral lobule dysfunction in the frontal lobes (figure 10.4). We shall return shortly to the frontal lobes to

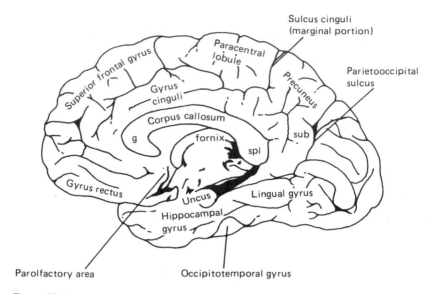

Figure 10.4
Medial surface of the right cerebral hemisphere showing the frontal lobes. Note, particularly, the paracentral lobule. (From Truex 1959)

analyze the organization of levels in the brain and the interaction of psychological and neural systems levels.

We may conclude that critical emotional-vegetative-social functions of the self are localized to the frontal lobes. Consequently frontal lobe systems are also involved in functions that contribute to subjective awareness and existence of the self. Further, it appears that the self represents an integration of functions that are distributed in multiple areas of the brain. The self, too, is modular functionally and physically. We have now localized some component parts of the self in discrete brain areas. The functions described serve to distinguish self from not self, monitor the physical state of the self, locate the self in space, and define the self in the social context. To complement the picture, can we now locate the self in time by identifying those faculties that endow the self with ontologic continuity? This task is far more difficult than those already discussed since the relevant database is far smaller and localization has been problematic. Nevertheless, a number of important clinical observations have been made in this sphere. Our goal is simply to determine whether there is evidence for a physical basis for this putative temporal faculty.

In fact, a variety of neurologic syndromes result in loss or impairment of the temporal continuity of the sense of self. One well-recognized example is the postconcussion syndrome (Haymaker 1969). Patients who receive a blow to the head with loss of conciousness frequently experience retrograde amnesia; they cannot remember events—the experiences that the self had immediately preceding and including the trauma. Over time, memory for this period is gradually filled in, with complete recovery. During the amnesic phase, however, that circumscribed history of the self is lost. While the precise locus of the deficit in the brain has not yet been identified, it is clear to all observers that the amnesia is based on physical disruption of critical brain processes. Moreover, the deficit is specific for memory and does not involve other mental faculties.

Another well-delineated though poorly localized syndrome is that of transient global amnesia (Fisher and Adams 1964). This disorder, due to decreased blood flow to the brain, results in the sudden onset of near-total disorientation of the self due to a virtually complete loss of recent memory (for example, see Shuttleworth and Wise 1973). Patients typically do not know how they got where they are, why they are there, or where they are going. The confusion appears to be based totally on the loss of memory for recent events and is thereby similar in kind to the postconcussion syndrome. Unlike the latter ill-localized disorder, however, transient global amnesia has been attributed to ischemia of the medial temporal lobe (Shuttleworth and Wise 1973), involving presumably the hippocampus. Once again, then, loss of the continuity of the self in time is attributable to pathophysiological brain mechanisms.

One final example of a very different type may round out our picture of the sense of self in time. The classic patient, H. M., underwent bilateral temporal lobe removal, with consequent removal of the hippocampi, to treat intractable epilepsy. The extensive studies of Milner and colleagues of this patient documented profound orthograde amnesia consequent to surgery (1959, 1962, 1970). H. M. is unable to lay down new memories and as a result requires chronic care. This is an instance of the self living in an eternal present, unable to form an ongoing subjective history.

These very different abnormalities indicate that the sense of self in time is based on underlying brain mechanisms. Viewed in conjunction with the foregoing clinical observations, a general conception of the organization of the self emerges. Most generally, it is apparent that subjective awareness and the sense of self are composed of discrete faculties on the psychological level. Further, these faculties are localized to different brain areas and probably to different neural systems within the brain. The self is an aggregate of component parts that are distributed in many brain areas, not a unitary entity. Contrary to intuitive, subjective impression, the self, too, is modular.

We can even delineate some of the faculties that comprise the self. A subjective sense involves knowledge of what is me and not me in space. It recognizes the state of physical function of the subjective entity. Another component governs actions in the social context. And yet another faculty endows the self with continuity in time. It is quite clear that *self* and *subjective awareness* are terms that encompass a large number of psychological symbols. The self is not a single psychological symbol or function.

In summary, we have been able to begin defining the self at a high level, that of psychological function, and at a lower level, that of localization in specific brain areas. The overarching point is that all of the foregoing considerations place the self and subjective awareness squarely within the biological system under discussion. There is no need to step out of the system to locate the most complex of psychological phenomena. It may be useful to restate our tentative formulations in general terms before proceeding to more detailed analyses. As a minimum, the subjective sense of self is composed of the self in space, the self in time, and the social self. In turn, these psychologic functions can be localized to regions of the parietal, temporal and frontal lobes at the gross anatomical level, and presumably to neural subsystems therein. We are at least partially on our way to understanding the construction of high-level subjective function in the context of lower-level neural structure. Our mandate now requires analysis in greater detail to determine whether specific aspects of brain organization allow, indeed demand, reciprocal interactions of low and high levels in the subjective hierarchy. To approach this issue, we might analyze the functional organization of any of the foregoing brain areas. We examine the frontal lobes, since they are central to subjective awareness and the sense of self.

The Frontal Lobes and the Principle of Reciprocity

Are there anatomic and neurochemical substrates that can subserve multidirectional interactions among levels? More specifically, how could high levels in the subjective cycle reach down to alter lower levels? Do such statements as "I am anxious" or "I am hungry" make sense on the basis of frontal organization or function? Even provisional answers may provide insights into the most basic relations between brain and mind function.

We begin by identifying some of the functions served by the frontal lobes in greater detail before delineating lower-level mechanisms upon which these are based. While patients with frontal lesions do perform adequately on the more routine intelligence tests, they nevertheless exhibit characteristic cognitive and emotional deficits. For example, they have particular difficulty with so-called divergent thought processes in which there are multiple solutions to a problem, multiple correct answers to a question, and multiple views of an object, in contrast to convergent thought, which allows only a single correct response. Divergent thinking appears to be critical for creative thought processes. These patients also perform inadequately on delayed-comparison tests in which paired stimuli must be distinguished after a discrete temporal delay. Further, work in patients as well as experimental animals has revealed that the frontal lobes subserve recognition-memory tasks, that lesions result in perseveration, loss of inhibitions, and impaired associational learning (Milner and Petrides 1984).

"Broadly stated, the frontal lobes are essential for synthetic reasoning, abstract thought, and the organization of independent behaviors in time and space towards future goals. Initiative, creativity, attentiveness, personal feeling and world view are, of necessity, expressive of the frontal-lobe's contribution to behavior" (Goldman-Rakic 1984b).

How are we to understand such a complexity of functions? At the neural systems level, the reciprocity of frontal connections forms an obvious, necessary physical basis for these behavioral and mental capabilities. The frontal lobes both innervate and are innervated by the posterior parietal, prestriate, and temporal cortices and the brainstem locus coeruleus (for review, see Goldman-Rakic 1984a). It is apparent that frontal function is intimately related to analysis and long-term storage of somatosensory, visual, and auditory information and is closely associated with attention, arousal, and anxiety. The neural circuitry itself is organized to allow higher integrative functions to interact with lower functions and symbols in a reciprocal manner through well-characterized feedback connections.

Further, projections of the frontal lobes to the hypothalamus and limbic system permit frontal integration and regulation of emotional, sexual, and appetitive behaviors and related mental processes. Projection to the precentral cortex and striatum regulates motor behavior (Evarts et al. 1984).

What are some of the consequences of this organization in terms of our construct? The frontal-locus coeruleus interactions are of interest in the light of our previous discussions. The frontal lobes have long been known to play a critical role in awareness, attention, and social inhibitions and a suspected role in anxiety. The recently described reciprocal connections to the locus explain some of these associations. Activation of the locus, evoking the attention-arousal-anxiety complex, is simultaneously related to frontal cortex through locus-frontal projections. The frontal cortex, in turn, may endow the anxiety state with appropriate affect and visual, auditory, and somatosensory associations. Further, attendant activation or inactivation of frontal-locus projections may determine whether the locus is restimulated or inhibited. Since locus tyrosine hydroxylase is responsive to the level of impulse stimulation, the high-level frontal mental function will have had access to the lower-level molecules upon which locus and, by connection, frontal function is partially based. In other words, the very organization of the brain virtually guarantees that high-level psychological function and cerebral centers alter the lower "hardware" upon which function is based.

The realization that the frontal cortex receives a dense, noradrenergic locus innervation suggested to Goldman-Rakic that frontal dysfunction in the elderly might be rectified by noradrenergic replacement therapy. Indeed, treatment of aged monkeys with the alpha-receptor agonist clonidine markedly improved cognitive performance, and treatment with the antagonist, yohimbine, prevented the salutory effect (Goldman-Rakic 1984a). Consequently, low-level molecules influence mind just as high-level mind influences molecules.

It might be expected that the frontal cortex, with access to stored visual, auditory, and sensory information, and with projections to limbic structures, is capable of manipulating and integrating these lower-level symbols into high-level cognitive and psychological symbols. In fact, Goldman-Rakic and coworkers (1984) have discovered that adult monkeys with prefrontal lesions perform as poorly as human infants on Piaget's AB Stage IV Object Permanence Test, a traditional task used to assess cognitive development in infants. This and related tests require that the individual realize that an object exists in time and space when absent from view. This capacity appears to be necessary for the development of symbolic reasoning, a cornerstone of higher cognitive function. This is one example of the manner in which the frontal lobes use sensory representations stored in other areas of the brain to build higher-level symbols of cognition. The reciprocal frontal connections imply, in turn, that frontal activity can affect the stored sensory representations themselves. A great deal of additional work will be required to validate this contention.

Frontal-Dopaminergic Connections

To appreciate more fully the potential role of the frontal cortex in stress and in mental disease, innervation by other catecholaminergic fibers must be considered. The frontal lobes receive a rich dopaminergic innervation from the ventral mesencephalic tegmentum (VMT), which induces a slow depolarization, reducing the firing rate (figure 10.5). This effect is mediated by the stimulation of Type 1 dopamine receptors (D_1), located on the frontal neurons. Spontaneous discharge of the frontal cortical neurons or discharge elicited by stimulation of the innervating mediodorsal thalamic nucleus is inhibited by excitation of the VMT. In summary, the VMT inhibits the frontal cortical neurons (for review, see Glowinski et al. 1984). The relationship of frontal neurons to dopaminergic cells is more complicated than that described. Frontal neurons project to the subcortical nucleus **accumbens,** which in turn also receives a dopaminergic input from the ventral tegmental area. Extensive evidence derived from lesion experiments indicates that frontal neurons normally decrease dopamine turnover and sensitivity to dopamine in the accumbens. Conversely, dopamine

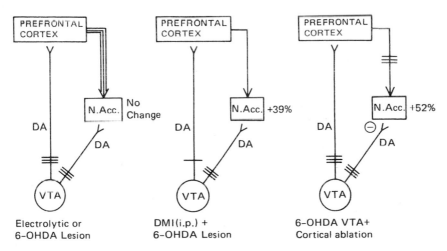

Figure 10.5
Frontal-subcortical dopaminergic connections. The schematic representations indicate the influence of the prefrontal cortex on the development of denervation supersensitivity of dopaminergic receptors in the rat nucleus accumbens. Denervation supersensitivity of dopamine receptor in the nucleus accumbens occurs only when mesocortico-prefrontal dopaminergic neurons are partially protected from lesions in the ventrotegmental area (VTA). Alternatively, the same sequence may result from a lesion of the prefrontal cortex following degeneration of the ascending dopaminergic neurons on the right. (From Glowinski 1984)

turnover and receptors are increased in accumbens after a selective lesion of the frontal dopamine neurons (for discussion, see Glowinski et al. 1984).

Extremely complex interactions among the mesencephalic VMT level, the frontal cortex level, and the subcortical accumbens level with respect to dopamine actions appear to regulate behavior. To understand the potential role of dopamine in mental dysfunction, it is necessary to consider the roles of cortical and subcortical dopaminergic connections (figure 10.5). (This anatomico-chemical feedback constitutes another type of continuous cycle or strange loop on a different level.)

With this complicated background, we now begin to characterize some of the behaviors associated with these dopaminergic pathways. The mesocortical neurons are particularly sensitive to stress. Dopamine turnover in the frontal cortex is increased dramatically, for example, by foot-shock stress, suggesting that this pathway is involved in the cortical reaction to environmental stress. Since the frontal cortex also innervates the locus coeruleus, a structure that may be involved in anxiety responses to stress, a complex feedback loop can be defined. Interestingly, benzodiazepines (such as valium), potent antianxiety agents, block activation of the mesocortical pathway by environmental stress. This may be a pivotal location for molecular therapy of reactions to stress. It certainly would be important to determine whether other forms of stress-reducing therapy affect the same neural pathway (Glowinski et al. 1984).

Tantalizing evidence hints that the VMT and its connections may play a role in mental diseases such as schizophrenia (Glowinski et al. 1984). Lesions of the VMT produce an extraordinary, permanent behavioral syndrome in the rat. Some of its components resemble symptoms in schizophrenia. The lesions result in locomotor hyperactivity, hyperreactivity to the environment, impairment of inhibition of previously learned responses and hoarding behavior, facilitation of approach learning and active avoidance, and increased distractibility. The severity of some abnormalities, such as locomotor hyperactivity, correlates with the degree of frontal dopaminergic denervation. Since decreased cortical dopamine turnover is associated with a rise in accumbens dopamine turnover and sensitivity and since dopamine antagonist, neuroleptic agents are effective in the treatment of schizophrenia, the disease may be associated with a complex of reduced frontocortical dopaminergic activity and increased subcortical dopaminergic activity. In other words, the efficacy of antipsychotic agents in schizophrenia may be due to predominant actions on the accumbens dopaminergic innervation. If VMT function is critical in the reaction to environmental stress and in the genesis of schizo-phrenic-like symptoms, we should want to know which neurons, in turn, regulate VMT activity. Considerable evidence indicates that the substance P-containing, habenulo-VMT tract activates the meso-frontal dopamine neurons. Substance P concentrations increase in the VMT in the stressed rat, and stimulation of the VMT dopamin-ergic neurons is blocked by injection of anti-SP antibodies (Thierry et al. 1984; Bannon et al. 1983). What factors govern the levels of sub-stance P?

Although we do not have a great deal of information regarding SP in the habenulo-VMT tract, the regulation of SP has been studied extensively in peripheral neurons. Moreover, the same transmitter characters appear to be similarly regulated in diverse neuronal pop-ulations. On this basis we can speculate that depolarization and trans-membrane sodium ion influx serve to decrease SP mRNA, and thus SP itself, in the habenular neurons. Conversely, decreased synaptic activation of the habenular neurons might be expected to increase SP levels. It will be of importance to determine whether, in fact, these predicted mechanisms underlie the changes in SP that are observed in stress. Regardless, it is apparent that environmental stimuli such as stress alter SP as well as dopamine metabolism in critical neural populations. A number of important implications should not be overlooked.

First, SP and dopamine participate in the stress response and pos-sibly in the pathogenesis of schizophrenic symptoms. Stated some-what differently, at least two entirely different transmitter systems play roles in the same mental states. On the other hand, derangement of very different transmitters may result in similar abnormalities at the behavioral level. While this is not terribly surprising, a priori, such explicit recognition should help us to eschew such naive concepts as "one transmitter, one disease," an approach that has characterized certain spheres of neuropsychopharmacology. A corollary of this re-alization indicates that mental diseases may be amenable to therapeu-tic approaches directed toward very different molecular loci. (This point has already been made when considering simultaneous dopa-minergic and anticholinergic therapy in Parkinson's disease.) In view of the variety of transmitters, co-localized, in series and in parallel, that underlie any given behavior or mental state, the profound pleio-tropy characteristic of neuropsychiatric disease is wholly expected.

Second, it is apparent that high-level behavior and mental state may affect multiple low-level transmitter systems simultaneously. For ex-ample, it is apparent that stress alters peptidergic, dopaminergic, and noradrenergic systems in different neural populations simultaneously.

It is these very systems in these very populations that mediate the responses of brain and mind to stress. Consequently, the complex array of high-level symbols that constitute a normal or abnormal mental state alters the function of manifold low-level neural systems and lower-level transmitters.

This complexity is certainly not unexpected considering the diverse array of signs and symptoms expressed in the archetypal disease, schizophrenia. As a bare minimum, auditory hallucinations, delusions, abnormal expression, and gross disorders of affect are part of this functional psychosis. Further, in catatonic schizophrenia, mutism, negativism, catalepsy (waxy flexibility of posturing), and staring into space may be observed (see, for example, Hearst et al. 1971; Morrison 1973; for overview, see McHugh 1982). We might anticipate that the disorder(s) may be generated by multiple abnormalities at the transmitter level and, indeed, by multiple disorders at very different levels. In fact, extensive evidence supports this contention.

It is now well recognized that there is a strong genetic component: 5 to 6 percent of siblings have the disease, and 40 to 50 percent of monozygotic twins of schizophrenic patients have schizophrenia, even if they have been raised separately (for review, see McHugh 1982). On an entirely different level, chronic amphetamine intoxication results in a syndrome that may be indistinguishable from schizophrenia behaviorally. Amphetamine releases norepinephrine and blocks reuptake inactivation of the transmitter. Similarly, alcohol withdrawal may result in a constellation of behaviors resembling the schizophrenic state. Moving to another level entirely, psychomotor epilepsy, resulting from a temporal or limbic irritative lesion, may also result in a schizophrenic syndrome. In summary, genetic, biochemical, and systems dysfunction may all contribute to the pathogenesis of schizophrenia. It is thus highly probable that abnormalities at multiple levels, causally interacting, result in the bizarre and tragic syndrome that we term schizophrenia.

The same genetic, transmitter, and systems levels that, when deranged, result in schizophrenia normally play critical roles in subjective awareness and the sense of self. For all the unknowns surrounding this baffling disease, none would deny that it is quintessentially a disorder of the sense of self. To summarize, whether we approach the problem of self and subjectivity from the perspective of normal or abnormal function, we are driven to specific brain areas, specific neural systems, and specific transmitters therein.

We now turn from a discussion of schizophrenia, one instance of a derangement of the levels that comprise the self, to reconsideration of normal frontal function. By appreciating the nature of anatomic connections of the frontal lobes, as examples of neocortical access to information on lower levels, and the important principle of reciprocity, we may begin to understand the manner in which the self can report on the state of itself. For example, the statement "I am anxious" can be conceived as the motor speech area reporting on the state of activity of locus-frontal and VMT-frontal connections, as a minimum. Similarly, the statement "I am hungry," among other possibilities, may reflect access of the frontal lobes to information in the lateral hypothalamic area (Grossman 1979). In the former case, we even have identified some of the lower-level molecular symbols upon which the neocortical reporting is based. These simplified examples illustrate a sense in which the self is simultaneously a part of, and apart from, lower-level affective and appetitive symbols. In addition, through reciprocal anatomic connections, the self may actually change lower levels and thereby alter the information upon which the speech area is reporting.

In summary, the continuous cycle, the continuous interaction of multiple levels, continually changes the self and its cognitive and emotional underpinnings. To remain with our paradigm, the frontal lobes, which consist of multiple levels and which deal with high-level psychological symbols, alter lower levels in the anatomic hierarchy, such as the locus, VMT, or lateral hypothalamus, which also consist of multiple levels. In turn, the lower anatomic levels directly or indirectly alter function of the frontal lobes. Levels within levels and cycles within cycles interact to form and mold the self.

We might well ask whether the principle of reciprocity, which permits the interaction of levels in the case of frontal function, applies to other brain regions and functions as well. In fact, this does appear to be the case. To cite a distant example, the subcortical relay nuclei that innervate the neocortex and limbic structures are also innervated by the same limbic areas (for example, see Kawamura and Chiba 1979; Swanson et al. 1974; Swanson and Hartman 1975; Swanson et al. 1986). Consequently the principle of anatomic reciprocity may be a basic organizing scheme of the brain. It may be concluded that multidirectional interactions among levels are fundamental to brain function and that higher-level regulation of lower-level symbols is widespread throughout the neuraxis. To recap, as in the case of frontal cognitive function, cortico-limbic emotional function is also characterized by interlevel interaction, and multiple interacting levels within a given anatomical locus.

The self, then, is a vast aggregate of functions distributed throughout the brain and even the entire neuraxis. Its component parts exist at multiple anatomic loci, and within these loci at multiple levels from neuronal population, to synaptic arrays, to symbolic molecules. Loci and levels are in continuous interaction constructing subjective reality.

Up to this point, we have restricted our considerations to interactions and events occurring within the individual nervous system. Recent observations suggest, however, that this view may be too restrictive. In a very important sense, discussions of "levels" must extend beyond the individual nervous system.

Interactions among Individuals

Extensive evidence indicates that interactions among individuals may exert profound effects on the individual nervous system. Perhaps the most dramatic documentation has derived from the field of reproductive physiology. The physiology of reproduction is under the direct control of the hypothalamo-pituitary axis, a part of the limbic system to which we have referred extensively.

A benchmark observation was made in 1971: college women living together developed menstrual synchrony (McClintock 1971). Subsequent experiments, designed to define underlying mechanisms, demonstrated that cohabiting female rats exhibit ovulatory synchrony. Further, females in isolation who are exposed to the odors of cycling female rats develop a synchrony of estrus, paralleling the cycling rats (McClintock 1978). Remarkably, community living in rodents or humans synchronizes ovulation. Moreover, in rats, and possibly humans, the synchrony results from exposure to an olfactory signal (McClintock 1981). "Levels" are inter- as well as intraindividual. Olfaction and the limbic system, as a minimum, are directly accessible to an external level—that of interanimal interaction. To the likely extent that ovulation affects and is affected by behavior and mental state, we may be sure that multiple loci in the nervous system, including the frontal lobes, are indirectly involved.

Since recent studies have defined the patterns of butyrates and squalenes that comprise the odors transmitting conspecific information in monkeys, it appears likely that the specific molecules eliciting ovulatory synchrony will soon be identified (Smith et al. 1985). **Even in the interanimal realm, then, neural levels of function, from mental state and behavior to molecules, constitute a critical organizing principle.** The importance of hierarchy in ecology and evolutionary biology, of course, has long been recognized.

Pursuing the role of the social level in the regulation of reproductive physiology, we next focus on a monogamous species, the common marmoset. While young marmosets still living with their mothers exhibited normal estrous cycles, the placement of five young females together in a peer group allowed only the dominant marmoset to ovulate (Abbott and Hearn 1978). Similarly, subordinate cotton-top tamarins suppress ovulation in a group (see Snowdon 1983). Removal of subordinate females and exposure to a male results in the initiation of ovulation within two weeks. The induced ovulation is suppressed when the female is reintroduced to a social context with a more dominant female.

These few examples from a large literature serve to illustrate the point: levels and cycles extend beyond the individual nervous system to involve the environment and other interacting individuals and nervous systems. Consequently, mental state, behavior, and resultant **interindividual molecular signals** affect levels and cycles within the individual nervous system. Each level can be defined in precise, physical terms. Further, in the sociobiological context, levels interact in a multidirectional fashion, obeying the dynamics described for cycles within individual nervous systems: higher social levels reach down to alter lower molecular levels, thereby changing social behavior itself.

In a broader sense, we may wonder whether continuous cycles represent an organizing principle applicable to life at all levels from single cells interacting with each other and the environment, to lower metazoa, to all higher forms acting singly and in social organizations. In the end, comprehensive descriptions of life systems may require definition of levels, from simple to complex, with clear delineation of the rules governing multidirectional interactions. The essence of life systems may involve the central fact that high levels continually transform the lower, elemental levels upon which the high levels are based. Appreciation, description, and analysis of this ubiquitous phenomenon may represent one of the fundamental tasks of the life sciences.

Glossary

Aboutness   Representation in the brain that allows intrinsic information to refer to external reality.

Acetylcholine   An excitatory amine transmitter used by subpopulations of neurons throughout the nervous system. The transmitter is synthesized by the enzyme choline acetyltransferase from acetyl coenzyme A and choline and is metabolized by the enzyme acetylcholinesterase.

Adrenal gland   A neuroendocrine organ, lying superior to the kidneys bilaterally, that is composed of the outer cortex, which secretes steroid hormones, and an inner medulla, which secretes epinephrine and norepinephrine. Adrenal steroids consist of glucocorticoids, which regulate intermediary metabolism, and mineralocorticoids, which regulate salt and water balance. Adrenal steroids and catecholamines participate in the stress response.

Affective disorders   Diseases characterized by derangements of mood and emotion such as depression and manic-depressive disorder.

Agnosias   Disorders of naming that result from cortical disconnection.

Alexia   Pathologic inability to read.

Alzheimer's Disease   A middle- to late-life degenerative neurologic disease of unknown etiology that results in the progressive death of multiple brain neuronal populations with profound cognitive impairment. The early degeneration of basal forebrain cholinergic neurons is thought to contribute to prominent memory deficits.

Amnesia   Memory deficit.

Amnesia, orthograde   Inability to form new memories normally.

Amnesia, retrograde   Defective memory for the past.

Amnesia, transient global   Temporary retrograde amnesia for all events, thought to result from decreased blood flow (ischemia) to the medial temporal lobes.

Amphetamines   A class of pharmacologic agents that release catecholamines from nerve terminals and inhibit the high-affinity uptake, inactivation of the amines. Amphetamine overdose may elicit a paranoid psychosis.

Amygdala   Group of neuronal nuclei in the dorsomedial temporal lobe bilaterally that subserve informational learning in conjunction with the hippocampus.

Anosagnosia   Pathological denial of disease attributable to dysfunction of the nondominant parietal lobe.

Aphasia   A general term referring to language-processing dysfunction that results in abnormalities of speech reception or expression.

Aplysia californica   A marine mollusc that has been the subject of extensive studies on the mechanisms of conditioning and simple behaviors.

Apraxias   Difficulties performing skilled movements in the absence of primary motor or sensory abnormalities. For example, certain patients may be unable to dress, although their primary sensorimotor function is normal.

Athetosis   Hyperkinetic movement disorder characterized by sinuous movements of the distal aspects of the limbs. May accompany chorea.

Auditory   Pertaining to the sense of hearing.

Autonomic nervous system   The sympathetic and parasympathetic subdivisions, which, in concert, regulate vegetative functions, including those governed by cardiovascular, respiratory, and gastrointestinal systems. While the generic term is frequently used to denote peripheral neurons of the system, central autonomic mechanisms govern peripheral autonomic function.

Autoreceptors   Receptors located on the membrane of afferent neurons that bind transmitter released by the same neuron, altering function. Autoreceptor activation commonly changes the subsequent release of the same or of a co-localized transmitter.

Axonal transport   The processes through which molecules and particulate matter are carried to different regions of the neuron. Orthograde transport, for example, carries molecules from the cell body to nerve terminals in targets, whereas retrograde transport carries molecules from terminals to cell body.

B_{max} A measure of the total number of receptors in a tissue, defined kinetically.

Basal forebrain cholinergic neurons   An extended group of neuronal nuclei at the base of the brain that innervate multiple cerebrocortical areas and utilize acetylcholine as a neurotransmitter. The neurons have been implicated in memory function.

Brainstem   The portion of the brain, composed of the medulla oblongata, the pons, and the midbrain, that governs a variety of vegetative functions and contains sensory and motor fibers of passage.

Broca's area   Area in the dominant frontal lobe that executes speech and that, when deranged, results in motor aphasia.

Catalysis   Enzymatic conversion of substrates to products.

Catecholamine   A family of neurotransmitters used by the sympathetic nervous system peripherally and by a number of brain systems, including the locus coeruleus (arousal and attention), the substantia nigra (which degenerates in Parkinson's disease), and the meso-cortical/subcortical (?deranged in schizophrenia) systems. The amines are also hormones elaborated by the adrenal medulla. Catecholamines are defined chemically as 3,4-dihydroxy derivatives of phenylethylamines. Prominent members include dopamine, norepinephrine, and epinephrine.

Cell adhesion molecules   Specific molecules expressed on the cell surface that mediate cell-cell interactions, such as selective adhesivity.

Cell cycle   The period between divisions of a cell, subdivided into the phases G1, S, G2, and M.

Cerebellum   That part of the brain lying superior to the fourth ventricle and brainstem that governs coordination of motor function and the orientation of the body in space.

Cerebral cortex   The layered mantle of neurons covering the hemispheres on their external, convex surfaces. The cortex subserves a variety of functions, including cognition.

Chemotaxis   Attraction to or repulsion of cells by specific molecules.

Choline acetyltransferase   The enzyme that catalyzes the synthesis of acetylcholine from choline and acetyl CoA.

Cholinergic   Referring to the use or expression of acetylcholine.

Chorea   Hyperkinetic movement disorder characterized by rapid, adventitious movements involving the proximal musculature. The disorder occurs in a variety of illnesses, including Huntington's disease, some forms of acute rheumatic fever, and complications of pregnancy.

Combinatorial strategy   Use of a limited series of elements to generate a large number of unique aggregates, or combinations.

Complementary DNA (cDNA)   DNA sequence synthesized in the laboratory from a specific cellular messenger RNA.

Conditioning, classical   Process of association between two stimuli, a conditioned and an unconditioned stimulus, resulting in the appearance of a conditioned response.

Conditioning, instrumental   Process of association between the response of an organism and a reinforcing stimulus.

Conformation, molecular   The structure of a molecule in three-dimensional space; tertiary structure of a molecule. The conformation of a protein is dictated by the primary structure, the sequence of amino acids that comprise the molecule.

Connectionism   A computational approach to cognition in which knowledge is thought to exist in the pattern and strength of connections among (neural) elements, such that learning consists of alteration of connections. Also termed *parallel distributed processing*.

Consensus sequence   A prototypical sequence of nucleotides that encodes a specific function, for example, the sequence that binds specific signal proteins.

Corpus callosum   Massive fiber tract that interconnects the two cerebral hemispheres, mediating information transfer.

Cyclic AMP   (3', 5'-adenosine monophosphate) A classic intracellular second messenger that transduces receptor binding into altered cellular function, commonly by phosphorylating cellular proteins. The molecule consists of phosphate groups linked to the ribose moiety.

Dendrites   Branched processes that are classically thought to conduct impulses to the neuronal cell body and that serve to integrate and summate spatiotemporally diverse inputs.

Developmental cell death   The normal ontogenetic process in which 50 to 80 percent of cells die in virtually all organ systems, including the nervous system.

Dictyostelium   The slime mold that undergoes different stages of cell aggregation during development, constituting a popular model for cell-cell interactions and ontogeny.

Disconnection syndromes   Neurologic disorders in which the receptive language (Wernicke's) area is deprived of normal sensory input, resulting in bizarre behavioral dissociations.

Dominant hemisphere   The cerebral hemisphere that processes language; the left hemisphere in most right-handed people.

Dopamine   The catecholamine transmitter used by substantia nigra neurons in the midbrain that regulate aspects of motor function. Dopaminergic deficits result in Parkinsonian signs and symptoms.

Electrochemical coding   Release of different and unique combinations of neurotransmitters by neurons in response to different frequencies and patterns of electical impulse activity.

Endorphins   Endogenous opiate peptides that exert analgesic actions and also affect the cardiovascular system.

Enkephalin   The basic peptide structure that confers opiate-like biologic activity and is incorporated into methionine-enkephalin, leucine-enkephalin, and endorphins. The enkephalins are synthesized as part of parent proenkephalin pro-molecules.

Enzyme   A molecule that increases the rate of a chemical reaction by orders of magnitude, converting substrates into products, without being permanently altered itself. While enzymes are generally proteins, recent work indicates that ribonucleic acids (RNAs) may also exhibit enzymatic (catalytic) activity.

Enzyme activation   Increased (catalytic) activity of an enzyme due to stimulation of preexistent enzyme molecules, in contrast to an increase in molecule number.

Enzyme induction   Increased enzyme molecule number, generally due to an increase in the rate of synthesis of the enzyme, commonly associated with a consequent rise in activity. In a formal sense, steady-state number may also increase due to a decrease in the rate of breakdown or decay.

Epigenetic   Pertaining to extragenomic factors. Epigenetic influences refer to signals originating outside the gene(s) of the subject cell or cells.

Epilepsy   A group of cerebrocortical disorders characterized by the convulsive, synchronous electrical discharge of cortical neurons that may result in overt seizures and loss of consciousness.

Epilepsy, psychomotor   Seizure disorders manifested by paroxysmal disturbances of behavior generally attributable to temporal lobe epilepsy.

Epinephrine   The predominant catecholamine elaborated by the adrenal medulla, mediating the stress response and mobilization for emergency. Epinephrine also is a transmitter used by a number of brainstem neuronal populations that regulate cardiovascular function.

Etiology   The causative agent of a disease.

Exon   A segment of an interrupted gene that is encoded in the processed messenger RNA product.

Frontal lobe   The most anterior of the cerebral lobes, it subserves motor function and synthetic reasoning and plays a major role in affective behavior.

Functionalism   The view that cognition, mentality, and neuropsychiatric function can be implemented by a variety of possible structures, only one of which is the brain as we know it.

G proteins   Nearly ubiquitous guanosine triphosphate binding proteins that transduce the activation of multiple receptor subtypes into cellular information.

Gene   Unit of the hereditary DNA macromolecule that normally encodes a biologically functional protein product.

Gene family   A closely related group of genes that encode proteins exhibiting amino acid sequence similarities. A gene family may arise evolutionarily through duplication of a primordial gene.

Gene product   In generic terms, the protein or messenger RNA encoded by a gene.

Genome   A generic term referring to the aggregate genetic material of an organism.

Glia   Nonneuronal cells in the nervous system that provide support, elaborate growth cues, terminate the actions of some transmitters, and serve multiple functions that are still being defined. Glia comprise several cell types, including astrocytes, oligodendroglia, and microglia.

Glucocorticoids   Steroid hormones that are elaborated by the adrenal cortex and that participate in normal metabolism and in stress responses. The hormones appear to act directly on neuronal populations, including those in areas of the cerebral cortex.

Growth factor   A molecule that regulates cell division (mitosis), whether derived from distant (endocrine), proximate (paracrine), or the same (autocrine) cells.

Gustatory   Pertaining to the sense of taste.

Habituation   Decreased efficacy of synaptic conduction consequent to repeated exposure to a stimulus.

Hardware   In neuroscience, by analogy with computer science, all elements that comprise the physical structure of the nervous system.

Hertz (Hz)   A measure of impulse frequency; 1 Hz = 1/second.

Hierarchy   A series of rank order.

Hippocampal formation   Cortical part of the olfactory system, located on the medial aspect of the temporal lobe, and consisting most prominently of the fimbria, hippocampus proper, the dentate gyrus, subiculum, and hippocampal gyrus. The formation has been implicated in memory function and has been employed extensively to study long-term potentiation.

Hypophysectomy   Removal of the pituitary, or master endocrine gland, commonly surgically.

Hypothalamus   The dense aggregation of neuronal subpopulations at the base of the brain, in the wall of the third ventricle extending from optic chiasm to mammillary bodies, that governs autonomic and visceral functions, including endocrine secretion, water balance, intermediary metabolism, temperature regulation, sexuality, appetite, and emotional behavior.

Inferior parietal lobule   A cortical association area lying at the junction of visual, auditory, and somesthetic sensory areas, which is the location of Wernicke's receptive language area.

Instantiation   In neuroscience and psychology, the implementation of mental function by structure.

Instruction   In the extreme view, isomorphic transfer of information from environment to organism or cell. Contrast with *selection*.

Interpreter   A cognitive agent in the dominant cerebral hemisphere that appears to elaborate hypotheses and explanations, bringing order and pattern to internal and external reality.

Intron   A segment of an interrupted gene transcribed into messenger RNA but subsequently excised during messenger RNA processing. Consequently, introns do not encode the final protein product.

Ion channel   A large molecule, or group of molecular subunits, inserted in the cell membrane, that forms a conduit for specific, small, electrically charged molecules. Passage of charged molecules may be regulated by voltage or neurotransmitter, as examples.

K_d A measure of the affinity of a receptor for a signal molecule, defined kinetically.

Kinase   An enzyme that catalyzes the transfer of a phosphate group to specific proteins, thereby altering structure and function.

Lesch-Nyhan syndrome   A genetic disorder affecting male children that is characterized by mental retardation, self-mutilation, choreoathetosis, and spasticity and is associated with a defect in the enzyme hypoxanthine phosphoribosyltransferase.

Limbic system   In classical neuroanatomy, the limbic lobe of Broca, consisting of the cingulate gyrus, isthmus, hippocampal gyrus and uncus, and the underlying subcortical cell nuclei, that regulates autonomic and visceral functions and aspects of behavior. Often regarded as a primitive system that governs instinctual activity.

Locus coeruleus   A group of approximately fourteen hundred noradrenergic neurons located in the rostral pons bilaterally that innervate the cerebral cortex, cerebellar cortex, and spinal cord. The locus is thought to mediate arousal, attention, and, potentially, forms of anxiety.

Long-term potentiation   Persistent strengthening of synaptic efficacy elicited by coincident electrical activation of different incoming neural pathways to the same nerve process.

Medial septal nucleus   A subdivision of the basal forebrain neuronal system that innervates the hippocampus and has been implicated in spatial memory.

Memory   In the context of this book, a generic phenomenon referring to the relatively long-term storage of information in a specific, precise manner.

Memory, procedural   Recall for nonrepresentational information, including motor skills such as bike riding.

Mesencephalon   The midbrain, lying between the pons and diencephalon, that contains the substantia nigra, certain cranial nerve nuclei, and sensorimotor fibers of passage.

Messenger RNA   The molecular intermediate, elaborated by genes, that serves as the template for synthesis of specific proteins in the cytoplasm.

Module, mental   A unit of cognitive function that constitutes a component of an integrated mental faculty. In one particular example, apparently unified visual experience consists of separate processing of color, motion, and depth perception.

Monera   Protozoan organisms having no defined nucleus.

Motor neuron disease   A progressive mid- to late-life degenerative neurologic disease in which primary motor neurons in the spinal cord and their afferents in the cerebral cortex degenerate, leading to paralysis, spasticity, and death due to respiratory compromise. Some forms are known as Lou Gehrig's disease.

Neocortex   The nonolfactory cerebral cortex that increases in size from reptiles to mammals and humans and subserves a variety of higher integrative functions.

Nerve growth factor   A trophic protein elaborated by targets and possibly glia that is required for the normal survival and function of peripheral sympathetic and sensory neurons and basal forebrain cholinergic neurons. Effects on other brain populations are under intense investigation.

Neuroleptic agents   Antipsychotic drugs, used to treat the psychoses, that exert beneficial effects on mood and disordered thought.

Neuron   The primary cellular element of the nervous system that conducts electrical impulse activity, communicates through neurotransmitter release, and stores information. The prototypical neuron consists of (1) dendrites, processes that receive signals, (2) the cell body or perikaryon in which the nucleus is located, and (3) a long axon, measuring meters in some cells, that terminates in the target tissue.

Neurotransmitters   Chemical signals that comunicate among neurons, and potentially between neurons and glia, resulting in such diverse effects as electrical impulse activity, altered gene expression, growth, and survival.

Norepinephrine   The sympathetic catecholamine in the peripheral nervous system and a transmitter used by the locus coeruleus in the brain.

Nucleus accumbens   A subcortical nucleus of neurons that may play a role in the pathogenesis of schizophrenia when deranged.

Nucleus basalis magnocellularis   A group of large neurons in the basal forebrain system that innervates the cerebral cortex and appears to play a role in memory function.

Nucleus of the diagonal band of Broca   A subdivision of the series of basal forebrain cholinergic nuclei that innervates regions of the cerebral cortex.

Olfactory system   Neural structures at the base of the brain that process odorant information and the motor responses thereto and that play a role in memory processing. The system includes the olfactory bulb, olfactory tract and striae, and the structures of the hippocampal formation.

Olivopontocerebellar atrophy   A mid- to late-life degenerative neurologic disease involving neurons in the brainstem and cerebellum, leading to muscle rigidity and cranial nerve abnormalities.

Paracentral lobule   Area on the medial aspect of the frontal lobe. Bilateral damage results in the frontal lobe bladder syndrome, in which patients urinate in public with apparent indifference to the impropriety of the act.

Parallel distributed processing   See Connectionism.

Parietal lobe, nondominant   Cerebral area lying posterior to the frontal lobe, anterior to the occipital lobe, and superomedial to the temporal lobe on the right side in most people. Lesions of the nondominant parietal lobe result in anosagnosia and left-sided (opposite) neglect, in addition to the cortical sensory syndrome, mild contralateral weakness, and contralateral visual impairment that occur with dysfunction of either parietal lobe.

Parkinson's disease   A middle- to late-life, progressive, degenerative neurologic disorder in which death of the substantia nigral dopaminergic neurons is accompanied by slowed movement (bradykinesia), muscle rigidity, masklike face, and stooped (festinating) gait.

Pathogenesis   The processes through which abnormal physiological mechanisms give rise to specific signs and symptoms.

Peptide   A string of amino acids, covalently linked through characteristic (peptide) chemical bonds.

Perikaryon   The cell body or soma of a neuron, which contains the nucleus.

Phenotypic expression   A generic term referring to the elaboration of specific gene products, including particular species of messenger RNA and the proteins they encode.

Phosphorylation   Enzymatic transfer of a phosphate chemical group to a biologically active molecule with alteration of structure and function.

Piaget's AB Stage IV Object Permanence Test   Traditional cognitive developmental test that requires the subject to realize that an object exists in time and space when absent from view.

Plasticity, neuronal   A generic term referring to mutability of structure and function, frequently induced by environmental experience.

Polyprotein   A polyfunctional protein that contains multiple biologically active molecules commonly released by proteolytic cleavage.

Porifera   Sponges.

Postconcussion syndrome   Symptom complex that includes temporary retrograde amnesia after loss of consciousness consequent to trauma.

Postsynaptic density (PSD)   A proteinaceous, disc-shaped structure apposed to the postsynaptic membrane of most chemical synapses. Transmitter receptors project into the synaptic cleft through the PSD, and the structure contains ion channels and articulates with motile cytoplasmic proteins, potentially allowing transduction of impulse activity into altered synaptic structure and function.

Posttranslational processing   All the reactions that modify the structure of a molecule subsequent to transcription and translation into a protein product. Such processes include proteolytic cleavage, phosphorylation, amidation, and glycosylation.

Prodynorphin One of the three endogenous opiate polyproteins. *See* proopiomelanocortin.

Prokaryotes Organisms devoid of nuclei.

Proopiomelanocortin (POMC) A polyprotein that contains ACTH (adrenocorticotropic hormone), endorphin, and MSHs (melanocyte stimulating hormones), which are released from the pituitary gland in response to environmental stress. POMC is also localized to other brain areas.

Protista A grouping containing the most primitive orders of plants and animals, including the Protophyta and Protozoa.

Receptor In general, a cell surface molecule that interacts with an extracellular signal molecule, with consequent conversion of the interaction into intracellular information that alters function. Alternatively, some receptors are located inside cells.

Receptors, nerve growth factor The cell surface molecule that binds nerve growth factor and mediates multifarious responses, including survival, hypertrophy, and increased expression of multiple gene products. The high-affinity ($K_d = 10^{-11}$ M), biologically active receptor and the low-affinity ($K_d = 10^{-9}$ M) forms appear to be encoded by a single gene.

Reductionism In neuroscience, the general view that mind function is ultimately explicable in terms of brain structure and function.

Restriction mapping Localization of sites on DNA that are cleaved by a group of (restriction) enzymes. Each enzyme cleaves at a specfic site, defined by nucleic acid sequence, yielding a characteristic DNA fragment that may be used for identification.

Ribosome A cytoplasmic organelle that translates messenger RNA into a protein product.

S phase The phase of the cell cycle during which DNA synthesis occurs.

Schizophrenia A group of major psychotic illnesses characterized by disordered thought, delusions, hallucinations, and disturbances of affect.

Selection Process through which the environment chooses among preexistent biologic mechnanisms or structures. Contrast with *instruction*.

Self The composite of neurocognitive faculties and modules that comprise subjective awareness.

Semantics In biology, the meaning of a symbol or symbol sets in terms of environmental representation and physiological effects.

Sensitization Increased (synaptic) response to a stimulus, generally attributable to exposure to a noxious stimulus.

Septohippocampal system Part of the basal forebrain-cortical system that plays a critical role in contextual-spatial memory.

Serotonin   An indoleamine transmitter derived from dietary tryptophan that is localized to brainstem raphé neurons, which appear to play a role in sleep.

Software   In neuroscience, by analogy with computer science, the functional program that dictates particular operations in the nervous system.

Somatosensory   Pertaining to general body sensations such as pain, touch, and position senses.

Southern blot   Transfer of denatured DNA from gel to a filter for hybridization with a complementary DNA or RNA.

Spatial memory, contextual   Recall that codes for position, location, and orientation in space in the context of such functions as body movement and head orientation. The hippocampus is thought to subserve this complex, integrated function.

Split brain   Brain in which the main connections between the cerebral hemispheres, the corpus callosum, and anterior commissure have been surgically transected. The procedure has been employed in intractable epilepsy to prevent the spread of abnormal electrical discharge from one hemisphere to the other.

Stress   A generic term referring to physiologic responses to perceived environmental threat or emergency. The stress response is thought to be mediated by a variety of neurohumoral mechanisms, including the concerted action of the limbic system, the central and peripheral autonomic systems, and the adrenal gland.

Striatum   The caudate, putamen, and globus pallidus, lying in the depths of the cerebral white matter, which regulate motor coordination and motor programs. The striatum is innervated by the substantia nigra, thalamus, and regions of the motor cortex and, in turn, innervates the hypothalamus, subthalamus, thalamus, red nucleus, and a number of motor nuclei.

Substance P   A putative peptide, excitatory transmitter that is localized to multiple subpopulations, including sensory and sympathetic neurons. The peptide contains 11 amino acids and is synthesized as part of a larger parent molecule, preprotachykinin, which also may contain the peptide transmitter NKA (substance K).

Substantia nigra   The large aggregates of neurons lying in the base of the midbrain bilaterally, which contain the dopaminergic cells of the pars compacta that innervate the striatum. The dopaminergic neurons regulate motor function and coordination and degenerate in Parkinson's disease.

Surface adhesion molecules   Molecules localized to the extracellular space that mediate specific interactions with selective cell types, such as selective adhesivity.

Symbol   In biological systems, a representational structure that participates in the on-going operation of the system itself.

Sympathetic nervous system   A division of the peripheral autonomic system distributed throughout the body that consists of afferent cholinergic neurons and efferent noradrenergic (norepinephrine-containing) neurons. In general terms, the system regulates multiple vegetative functions, including the cardiorespiratory and gastrointestinal systems, and mediates the so-called fight-or-flight physiologic-behavioral repertoire.

Synapse   The specialized junction between neurons through which communication occurs.

Syntax   Rules that define relations among elements of a system.

Temporal amplification   Conversion of a brief environmental stimulus into relatively long-lasting neural information.

Tertiary structure   See Conformation.

Tetrahymena pyriformis   A unicellular ciliate (protozoan) resembling a paramecium that contains a number of transmitter gene products.

Transcription, gene   The complex of processes that comprise synthesis of messenger RNA from the DNA genetic code. In turn, messenger RNA is translated into protein product that functions in the cell.

Transduction   In biological systems, conversion of one form of information into another.

Translation   Synthesis of protein from specific, encoding messenger RNA.

Trophic factor   A molecule that supports survival of a cellular population.

Tyrosine hydroxylase   The rate-limiting enzyme in catecholamine biosynthesis, which consequently regulates the production of dopamine, norepinephrine, and epinephrine.

Ventral mesencephalic tegmentum   Area of the midbrain that contains dopaminergic neurons, which project to frontal cortical neurons and to neurons of the nucleus accumbens. These dopaminergic systems, and their projection areas, may play roles in the pathogenesis of schizophreniform symptoms.

Vesicles   Membrane-bound granules in nerve terminals that store neurotransmitter and release the molecules in response to impulse activity.

Werdnig-Hoffman's disease   A congenital form of motor neuron disease.

Wernicke's area   The receptive language area located at the junction of the dominant temporal, parietal, and occipital lobes, which, when deranged, results in sensory aphasia.

Bibliography

Abbott, D. H., and Hearn, J. P. 1978. Physical hormonal and behavioural aspects of sexual development in the marmoset monkey. Callithrix jacchus. J. Reprod. Fertil. 53:155–166.

Adams, R. D. 1962. Disorders of nervous function. In *Principles of Internal Medicine*, T. H. Harrison, R. D. Adams, I. L. Bennet, W. H. Resnik, G. W. Thorn, and M. M. Wintrobe (eds.), pp. 235–415. Blakiston Division, McGraw-Hill, New York.

Adler, R., Landa, K. B., Manthorpe, M., and Varon, S. 1979. Cholinergic neuronotrophic factors: Intraocular distribution of trophic activity for ciliary neurons. Science 204:1434–1436.

Ahlquist, R. P. 1948. A study of the adrenotropic receptors. Amer. J. Physiol. 153:586–600.

Akil, H., Watson, S. J., Young, E., Lewis, M. E., Khachaturian, H., and Walker, J. M. 1984. Endogenous opioids: Biology and function. Ann. Rev. Neurosci. 7:223–255.

Andersen, P., Sundberg, S. H., Swann, J. W., and Wigstrom, H. 1980. Possible mechanisms for long-lasting potentiation of synaptic transmission in hippocampal slices from guinea pigs. J. Physiol. Lond. 302:463–482.

Andreoli, T. E. 1982. Antidiuretic hormone. In *Textbook of Medicine*, Wyngaarden, J. B. and Smith, L. H., Jr. (eds.), pp. 1192–1195. W. B. Saunders Co., Philadelphia.

Angeletti, R. H., and Bradshaw, R. A. 1971. Nerve growth factor from mouse submaxillary gland: Amino acid sequence. Proc. Natl. Acad. Sci. USA 68:2417–2420.

Angeletti, R. H., Bradshaw, R. A., and Wade, R. D. 1971. Subunit structure and amino acid composition of mouse submaxillary gland nerve growth factor. Biochemistry 10:463–469.

Angeletti, R. H., Mercanti, D., and Bradshaw, R. A. 1973a. Amino acid sequences of mouse 2.5S nerve growth factor. I. Isolation and characterization of the soluble tryptic and chymotryptic peptides. Biochemistry 12.90–99.

Angeletti, R. H., Hermodson, M. A., and Bradshaw, R. A. 1973b. Amino acid sequences of mouse 2.5S nerve growth factor. II. Isolation and characterization of the thermolytic and peptic peptides and the complete covalent structure. Biochemistry 12:90–99.

Aston-Jones, G., and Bloom, F. E. 1981a. Activity of norepinephrine-containing locus coeruleus neurons in behaving rats anticipates fluctuations in the sleep-waking cycle. J. Neurosci. 1:876–886.

Aston-Jones, G., and Bloom, F. E. 1981b. Norepinephrine-containing locus coeruleus neurons in behaving rats exhibit pronounced responses to non-noxious environmental stimuli. J. Neurosci. 1:887–900.

Ayer-LeLievre, C., Olson, L., Ebendal, T., Seiger, A., and Persson, H. 1988. Expression of the β-nerve growth factor gene in hippocampal neurons. Science 240:1339–1341.

Bailey, C. 1989. Time course of structural changes at identified sensory neuron synapses during long-term sensitization in aplysia. J. Neurobiol. 9:1774–1780.

Bannon, M. J., Elliott, P. J., Alpart, J. E., Goedert, M., Iversen, S. D., and Iversen, L. L. 1983. Role of endogenous substance P in stress-induced activation of mesocortical dopamine neurones. Nature (Lond.) 306:791–792.

Barbin, G., Manthorpe, M., and Varon, S. 1984. Purification of a new neurotrophic factor from mammalian brain. EMBO J. 1:549–553.

Bartfai, T., Iverfeldt, K., Brodin, E., and Ogren, S.-O. 1986. Functional consequences of coexistence of classical and peptide neurotransmitters. In Progress in Brain Research. T. Hokfelt, K. Fuxe, and B. Pernow (eds.), vol. 68, pp. 321–330. Elsevier Science Publishers B.V. (Biomedical Division), New York.

Bartus, R. T. 1978. Evidence for a direct cholinergic involvement in the scopolamine induced amnesia in monkeys: Effects of concurrent administration of physostigmine and methylphenidate with scopolamine. Pharmacol. Biochem. Behav. 9:833.

Bartus, R. T., and Johnson, H. R. 1976. Short-term memory in the Rhesus monkey: Disruption from the anticholinergic scopolamine. Pharmacol. Biochem. Behav. 5:39.

Bartus, R. T., Dean, R. L. III., Beer, B., and Lippa, A. S. 1982. The cholinergic hypothesis of geriatric memory dysfunction. Science 217:408–417.

Bear, M. F., Cooper, L. N. and Ebner, F. F. 1987. A physiological basis for a theory of synapse modification. Science 237:42–48.

Berger, T. W., and Thompson, R. F. 1978. Neuronal plasticity in the limbic system during classical conditioning of the rabbit nictitating membrane response. I. The hippocampus. Brain Res. 145:323–346.

Bernd, P., Martinez, H. J., Dreyfus, C. F., and Black, I. B. 1988. Localization of high-affinity and low-affinity nerve growth factor receptors in cultured rat basal forebrain. Neurosci. 26:121–129.

Biguet, N. F., Buda, M., Lamouroux, A., Samolyk, D., and Mallet, J. 1986. Time course of the changes of TH mRNA in rat brain and adrenal medulla after a single injection of reserpine. EMBO J. 5:287–291.

Birkmayer, W., and Hornykiewicz, O. 1961. O: Der L–3,4-Dioxyphenylalanin (DOPA)-Effekt bei der Parkinson-Akinese. Wien Klin. Wschr. 73:787–788.

Bjerre, B., Bjorklund, A., Mobley, W., and Rosengren, E. 1975a. Short- and long-term effects of nerve growth factor of the sympathetic nervous system in the adult mouse. Brain Res. 94:263–277.

Bjerre, B., Wiklund, L., and Edwards, D. C. 1975b. A study of the de- and regenerative changes in the sympathetic nervous system of the adult mouse after treatment with the antiserum to nerve growth factor. Brain Res. 92:257–278.

Black, I. B. 1975. Increased tyrosine hydroxylase activity in frontal cortex and cerebellum after reserpine. Brain Res. 95:170–176.

Black, I. B. 1982. Stages of neurotransmitter development in autonomic neurons. Science 215:1198–1204.

Black, I. B., Adler, J. E., Dreyfus, C. F., Friedman, W. F., LaGamma, E. F., and Roach, A. H. 1987. Biochemistry of information storage in the nervous system. Science. 236:1263–1268.

Black, I. B., and Reis, D. J. 1975. Ontogeny of the induction of tyrosine hydroxylase by reserpine in the superior cervical ganglion, nucleus locus coeruleus and adrenal gland. Brain Res. 84:269–278.

Black, I. B., Chikaraishi, D. M., and Lewis, E. J. 1985. Trans-synaptic increase in RNA coding for tyrosine hydroxylase in a rat sympathetic ganglion. Brain Res. 339:151–153.

Black, I. B., Hendry, I. A., and Iversen, L. L. 1971. Differences in the regulation of tyrosine hydroxylase and DOPA decarboxylase in sympathetic ganglia and adrenals. Nature New Biol. *231*:27–29.

Bliss, T. V. P., and Lomo, T. 1973. Long lasting potentiation of synaptic transmission in the dentate area of the anesthetized rabbit following stimulation of the perforant path. J. Physiol. Lond. *232*:331–356.

Blum, J. J. 1970. On the regulation of glycogen metabolism in tetrahymena. Arch. Biochem. Biophys. *137*:65.

Bohn, M. C., Kessler, J. A., Golightly, L., and Black, I. B. 1983. Appearance of enkephalin-immunoreactivity in rat adrenal medulla following treatment with nicotinic antagonists or reserpine. Cell Tiss. Res. *231*:469–479.

Bowen, D. M., Sims, N. R., Benton, J. S., Curzon, G., Davidson, A. N., Neary, D., and Thomas, D. J. 1981. Treatment of Alzheimer's disease, a cautionary note. N. Eng. J. Med. *305*:1016.

Bradshaw, R. A. 1978. Nerve growth factor. Ann. Rev. Biochem. *47*:191–216.

Branton, W. D., Phillips, H. S., and Jan, Y. N. 1986. The LHRH family of peptide messengers in the frog nervous system. In *Progress in Brain Research*, T. Hokfelt, K. Fuxe, and B. Pernow (eds.), vol. 68, pp. 205–215. Elsevier Science Publishers B.V. (Biomedical Division), New York.

Brodmann, K. 1908. Beitrage zur histologischen Lokalisation der Grosshirnrinde. VI. Mitteilung. Die Cortexgliederung des Menschen. J. Psychol. Neurol. *10*:231–246.

Brownstein, M. J., and Mezey, E. 1986. Multiple chemical messengers in hypothalamic magnocellular neurons. In *Progress in Brain Research*, T. Hokfelt, K. Fuxe, and B. Pernow (eds.), vol. 68, pp. 161–168. Elsevier Science Publishers B.V. (Biomedical Division), New York.

Brunso-Bechtold, J. K., and Hamburger, V. 1979. Retrograde transport of nerve growth factor in chicken embryo. Proc. Natl. Acad. Sci. USA *76*:1494–1496.

Buck, C. R., Martinez, H. J., Black, I. B., and Chao, M. V. 1987. Developmentally regulated expression of the nerve growth factor receptor gene in the periphery and brain. Proc. Natl. Acad. Sci. USA *84*:3060–3063.

Buck, C. R., Martinez, H. J., Chao, M. V., and Black, I. B. 1988. Differential expression of the nerve growth factor receptor gene in multiple brain areas. Devel. Br. Res. *44*:259–268.

Bullock, T. H. 1977. *Introduction to Nervous Systems*. W. H. Freeman, San Francisco.

Burnstock, G. 1986. Purines as cotransmitters in adrenergic and cholinergic neurones. In *Progress in Brain Research*. T. Hokfelt, K. Fuxe, and B. Pernow (eds.), vol. 68, pp. 193–203. Elsevier Science Publishers B.V. (Biomedical Division), New York.

Carlsson, A., Lindquist, M., Magnusson, T., and Waldeck, B. 1958. On the presence of 3-hydroxytyramine in brain. Science *127*:471.

Caskey, C. T. 1987. Disease diagnosis by recombinant DNA methods. Science *236*:1223–1229.

Cedarbaum, J., and Aghajanian, G. 1976. Noradrenergic neurons of the locus coeruleus: Inhibition by epinephrine and activation by the α-antagonist piperoxane. Brain Res. *112*:413–419.

Changeux, J.-P. 1985. *Neuronal Man*. Pantheon Books, New York.

Chao, M. V., Bothwell, M. A., Ross, A. H., Koprowski, H., Lanahan, A. A., Buck, C. R., and Sehgal, A. 1986. Gene transfer and molecular cloning of the human NGF receptor. Science *232*:518–521.

Chlatkowski, F. J., and Butcher, R. W. 1973. Subcellular distribution of adenyl cyclase and phosphodiesterase in acanthomoeba palestinensis. Biochem. Biophys. Acta. *309*:138.

Churchland, P. S. 1986. *Neurophilosophy*. MIT Press. Cambridge, MA.

Cohen, R. J., Ness, J. L., and Whiddon, S. M. 1980. Adenylate cyclase from phycomyces sporangiophore. Phytochem. *19*:1913.

Collingridge, G. L., Kehl, S. L., and McLennan, H. 1983. Excitatory amino acids in synaptic transmission in the Schaffer collateral-commissural pathway of the rat hippocampus. J. Physiol. Lond. *334*:33.

Comb, M., Herbert, E., and Crea, R. 1982. Partial characterization of the mRNA that codes for enkephalins in bovine adrenal medulla and human pheochromocytoma. Proc. Natl. Acad. Sci. USA *79*:360–364.

Comb, M., Rosen, H., and Herbert E. 1983. Structure of the human pro-enkephalin gene: Clustering of C_pG sequences and relationship to methylation. J. DNA *2* (3):278–290.

Cooper, J. R., Bloom, F. E., and Roth, R. H. 1982. *The Biochemical Basis of Neuropharmacology*. Oxford University Press, New York.

Cotzias, G. C., Papavasiliou, P. S., and Gelene, R. 1969. Modification of Parkinsonism—chronic treatment with L-Dopa. N. Eng. J. Med. *280*:337–345.

Cotzias, G. C., Van Woert, M. H., and Schiffer, L. M. 1967. Aromatic amino acids and modification of parkinsonism. New Eng. J. Med. *276*:374–379.

Cowan, W. M., Fawcett, J. W., O'Leary, D. D. M., and Stanfield, B. B. 1984. Regressive events in neurogenesis. Science *225*:1258–1265.

Coyle, J. T., Price, D. L., and DeLong, M. R. 1983. Alzheimer's disease: A disorder of cortical cholinergic innervation. Science *219*:1184–1190.

Crawley, J. N. 1985. Cholecystokinin potentiation of dopamine mediated behaviors in the nucleus accumbens. In *Neuronal Cholecystokinin*, J. J. Vanderhaeghen and J. N. Crawley (eds.), vol. 448, pp. 283–292. New York Academy of Sciences, New York.

Crawley, J. N., Stivers, J. A., Blumstein, L. K., and Paul, S. M. 1985. Cholecystokinin potentiates dopamine-mediated behaviors:evidence for modulation specific to a site of co-existence. J. Neurosci. *5*(8):1972–1983.

Darwin, C. 1859. *The Origin of Species*. Reprint. 1968, Penguin Books, New York.

De Ceccatty, M. P. 1974. The origin of the integrative systems: A change in view derived from research on Coelenterates and sponges. Persp. Biol. Med. *17*:379.

Denis-Donini, S. 1989. Expression of dopaminergic phenotypes in the mouse olfactory bulb induced by the calcitonin gene-related peptide. Nature *339*:701–703.

Devreotes, P. 1989. Dictyostelium discoideum: a model system for cell-cell interactions in development. Science *245*:1054–1058.

DiCicco-Bloom, E., and Black, I. B. 1988. Insulin growth factors regulate the mitotic cycle in cultured rat sympathetic neuroblasts. Proc. Natl. Acad. Sci. USA *85*:4066–4070.

Douglas, R. J., and Truncer, P. C. 1976. Parallel but independent effects of pentobarbital and scopolamine on hippocampus-related behavior. Behav. Biol. *18*:359–367.

Drachman, D., and Leavitt, J. 1974. Human memory and the cholinergic system. Arch. Neurol. (Chicago) *30*:113.

Dreyfus, C. F., Bernd, P., Martinez, H. J., Rubin, S. J., and Black, I. B. 1989. GABA-ergic and cholinergic neurons exhibit high-affinity nerve growth factor binding in rat basal forebrain. Exper. Neurol. *104*:181–185.

Dreyfus, C. F., Friedman, W. J., Markey, K. A., and Black, I. B. 1986. Depolarizing stimuli increase tyrosine hydroxylase in the mouse locus coeruleus in culture. Brain Res. *379*:216–222.

Dreyfus, C. F., Markey, K. A., Goldstein, M., and Black, I. B. 1983. Development of catecholaminergic phenotypic characters in the mouse locus coeruleus *in vivo* and in culture. Devel. Biol. *97*:48–58.

Dun, N. I., and Karczmar, A. G. 1979. Actions of substance P on sympathetic neurons. Neuropharmacologia *18*:215–218.

Ebendal, T., Larkfors, L., Lievre, C. A., Seiger, A., and Olson, L. 1983. New approaches to detect NGF-like activity in issues. Horm. Cell Regul. 9:361–376.

Ebendal, T. L., Olson, A., Seiger, A., and Hedlund, K. O. 1980. Nerve growth factors in the iris. Nature 288:25–28.

Eckerman, D. A., Gordon, W. A., Edwards, J. D., McPhail, R. C., and Gage, M. I. 1980. Effects of scopolamine, phenobarbital and amphetamine on radial arm maze performance in the rat. Physiol. Behav. 12:595–602.

Edelman, G. M. 1988. Topobiology: An Introduction to Molecular Embryology. Basic Books, New York.

Ehringer, H., and Hornykiewicz, O. 1960. Verteilung von Noradrenalin und Dopamin (3-hydroxytyramin) im Gehirn des Menschen und ihr Verhalten bei Erkrankungen des extrapyramidalen systems. Wien Klin. Wschr. 38:1236–1239.

Eichenbaum, H., and Cohen, N. J. 1988. Representation in the hippocampus: What do the neurons code? TINS 11:244–248.

Eichenbaum, H., Weiner, S. I., Shapiro, M., and Cohen, N. J. 1989. The organization of spatial coding in the hippocampus: A study of neural ensemble activity. J. of Neurosci. 9:2764–2775.

Elliot, R. R. 1905. The action of adrenaline. J. Physiol. (Lond.) 32:401–467.

Ernsberger, U., Sendtner, M., and Rohrer, H. 1989. Proliferation and differentiation of embryonic chick sympathetic neurons: Effects of ciliary neurotrophic factor. Neuron. 2:1275–1284.

Euler, U. S. von. 1959. Autonomic neuroeffector transmission. In Handbook of Physiology, p. 215, American Physiological Society, Washington, D.C.

Evarts, E. V., Kimura, M., Wurtz, R. H., and Hikosaka, O. 1984. Behavioral correlates of activity in basal ganglia neurons. TINS 7:447–453.

Fahn, S. 1982. The choreas. In Textbook of Medicine, J. B. Wyngaarden and L. H. Smith, Jr., (eds.), pp. 2029–2034. Saunders Co., Philadelphia.

Falck, B., Hillarp, N.-A., Thieme, G., and Thorpe, A. 1962. Fluorescence of catecholamines and related compounds condensed with formaldehyde. J. Histochem. Cytochem. 10:348–354.

Felsenfeld, G., and McGhee, J. 1982. Methylation and gene control. Nature (Lond.) 296:602–605.

Fischli, W., Goldstein, A., Hunkapiller, M., and Hood, L. E. 1982. Two "big" dynorphins from porcine pituitary. Life Sci. 31:1769–1772.

Fisher, C. M., and Adams, R. D. 1964. The transient global amnesic syndrome. Acta. Neurol. Scand. Suppl. 9, 40:7–82.

Flanagan, O. P., Jr. 1984. The Science of the Mind. MIT Press, Bradford Books, Cambridge, MA.

Flawia, M. M., and Torres, H. N. 1972. Activation of membrane-bound adenylate cyclase by glucagon in Neurospora crassa. Proc. Acad. Sci. USA 69:2870.

Fodor, J. 1979. The Language of Thought. Harvard University Press, Cambridge, MA.

Fodor, J. 1983. The Modularity of Mind. MIT Press, Bradford Books, Cambridge, MA.

Fodor, J. A., and Pylyshyn, Z. W. 1988. Connectionism and cognitive achitecture: a critical analysis. Cognition 28:3–71.

Franquinet, R., and Martelly, I. 1981. Effects of serotonin and catecholamines on RNA synthesis in planarians; in vitro and in vivo studies. Cell Diff. 10:201.

Fukuchi, I., Kato, S., Nakahiro, M., Uchida, S., Ishida, R., and Yoshida, H. 1987. Blockade of cholinergic receptors by an irreversible antagonist, propylbenzilylcholine mustard (PrBCM), in the rat cerebral cortex causes deficits in passive avoidance learning. Brain Res. 400:53–61.

Fuxe, K., Agnati, L., Benefenati, F., Cimmino, M., Algeri, S., Hokfelt, T., and Mutt, V. 1981. Modulation by cholecystokinin of ^{3}H-spiropendol binding in rat striatum:

evidence for increased affinity and reduction in number of binding sites. Acta Physiol. Scand. 113:567–569.

Gage, F. H., Wictorin, K., Fisher, W., Williams, L. R., Varon, S., and Bjorklund, A. 1986. Chronic intraventricular infusion of nerve growth factor (NGF) improves memory performance in cognitively impaired aged rats. Soc. Neurosci. Abstr. 12:1580.

Galaburda, A. M., LeMay, M., Kemper, T. L., and Geschwind, N. 1978. Right-left asymmetries in the brain. Science 199:852–856.

Gazzaniga, M. S. 1970. The Bisected Brain. Appleton-Century, Croft, New York.

Gazzaniga, M. S. 1985. The Social Brain. Basic Books, New York.

Gazzaniga, M. S. 1989. Organization of the human brain. Science 245:947–952.

Gazzaniga, M. S., and LeDoux, J. E. 1978. The Integrated Mind. Plenum, New York.

Geschwind, N. 1965. Disconnexion syndromes in animals and man. Brain 88:237–585.

Geschwind, N., and Levitsky, W. 1968. Human brain: Left-right Asymmetries in temporal speech region. Science 161:186.

Geula, C., and Mesulam, M. M. 1989. Cortical cholinergic fibers in aging and Alzheimer's disease: A morphometric study. Neurosci. 33:469–481.

Giorguieff, M. F., LeFloch, M. L., Westfall, T. C., and Glowinski, J. 1976. Nicotinic effect of acetylcholine on the release of newly synthesized [^{3}H] dopamine in rat striatal slices and cat caudate nucleus. Brain Res. 106:117–131.

Glowinski, J., Tassin, J. P., and Thierry, A. M. 1984. The mesocortico-prefrontal dopaminergic neurons. TINS 7:415–418.

Glucksman, A. 1951. Cell death in normal vertebrate ontogeny. Biol. Rev. 26:59–86.

Gnahn, H., Hefti, F., Heumann, R., Schwab, M. E., and Thoenen, H. 1983. NGF-mediated increase of choline acetyltransferase (ChAT) in the neonatal rat forebrain: Evidence for a physiological role of NGF in the brain. Dev. Brain Res. 9:45–52.

Goldman-Rakic, P. S. 1984a. Modular organization of prefrontal cortex. TINS 7:419–424.

Goldman-Rakic, P. S. 1984b. The frontal lobes: Uncharted provinces of the brain. TINS 7:425–429.

Goldstein, A., Fischli, W., Lowney, L. I., Hunkapiller, M., and Hood, L. 1981. Porcine pituitary dynorphin: Complete amino acid sequence of the biologically active heptadecapeptide. Proc. Natl. Acad. Sci. USA 78:7219–7223.

Goldstein, A., Tachibana, S., Lowney, L. I., Hunkapiller, M., and Hood, L. 1979. Dynorphin-(1–13), an extraordinarily potent opioid peptide. Proc. Natl. Acad. Sci. USA 76:6666–6667.

Goldstein, M., Bronaugh, R. L., Ebstein, B., and Roberge, C. 1976. Stimulation of tyrosine hydroxylase activity by cyclic AMP in synaptosomes and in soluble striatal enzyme preparations. Brain Res. 109:563–574.

Goodman, C. S., Pearson, K. G., and Heitler, W. J. 1979. Variability of identified neurons in grasshoppers. Comp. Biochem. Physiol. 64A:455–462.

Govoni, S., Hanbauer, I., Hexum, T. D., Yang, H.-Y.T., Kelley, G. D., and Costa, E. 1981. In vivo characterization of the mechanisms that secrete enkephalin-like peptides stored in dog adrenal medulla. Neuropharmacology 20:639–645.

Gray, T. S., and Morley, J. E. 1986. Neuropeptide Y: anatomical distribution and possible function in mammalian nervous system. Life Sciences 38:389–401.

Greene, L. A., and Shooter, E. M. 1980. The nerve growth factor: Biochemistry, synthesis, and mechanism of action. Ann. Rev. Neurosci. 3:353–402.

Greengard, P. 1976. Possible role for cyclic nucleotides and phosphorylated membrane proteins in postsynaptic actions of neurotransmitters. Nature 260:101–108.

Greenough, W. T. 1984. Structural correlates of information storage in the mammalian brain: A review and hypothesis. TINS 7:229–233.

Grene, M. 1987. Hierarchies in biology. American Scientist 75:504—510.

Grossman, S. P. 1979. The biology of motivation. Ann. Rev. Psychol. 30:209–242.

Gubler, H., Kilpatrick, D. L., Seeburg, P. H., Gage, L. P., and Udenfriend, S. 1981. Detection and partial characterization of proenkephalin mRNA. Proc. Natl. Acad. Sci. USA 78:5484–5487.

Hamburger, V., Brunso-Bechtold, J. K., and Yip, J. W. 1981. Neuronal death in the spinal ganglia of the chick embryo and its reduction by nerve growth factor. J. Neurosci. 1:60–71.

Hamburger, V., and Levi-Montalcini, R. 1949. Proliferation, differentiation and degeneration in the spinal ganglia of the chick embryo under normal and experimental conditions. J. Exp. Zool. 111:457–502.

Hanley, M. R. 1989a. Mitogenic neurotransmitters. Nature 340:97.

Hanley, M. R. 1989b. Peptide regulatory factors in the nervous system. Lancet 1:1373–1376.

Harrison, T. H., Adams, R. D., Bennett, I. L., Resnik, W. H., Thorn, G. W., and Wintrobe, M. M. 1962. Principle's of Internal Medicine, 4th ed. Blakiston Division, McGraw-Hill, New York.

Haymaker, W. 1969. Bing's Local Diagnosis in Neurological Diseases. C. V. Mosby Company, St. Louis.

Hearst, E. D., Munoz, R. A., and Fuason, V. B. 1971. Catatonia: Its diagnostic validity. Dis. Nerv. Syst. 32:453–456.

Hebb, D. O. 1949. The Organization of Behavior. Wiley, New York.

Hefti, F. 1986. Nerve growth factor promotes survival of septal cholinergic neurons after fimbrial transection. J. Neurosci. 6:2155–2162.

Hefti, F., Hartikka, J., and Bolger, M. B. 1986. Effect of thyroid hormone analogs on the activity of choline acetyltransferase in cultures of dissociated septal cell. Brain Res. 375:413–416.

Hefti, F., Hartikka, J., Eckenstein, F., Gnahn, H., Heumann, R., and Schwab, M. 1985. Nerve growth factor increases choline acetyltransferase but not survival or fiber outgrowth of cultured fetal septal cholinergic neurons. Neurosci. 14:55–68.

Hendry, I. A. 1977. The effect of the retrograde axonal transport of nerve growth factor on the morphology of adrenergic neurons. Brain Res. 134:213–223.

Hendry, I. A., Stach, R., and Herrup, K. 1974a. Characteristics of the retrograde axonal transport system for nerve growth factor in sympathetic nervous system. Brain Res. 82:117–128.

Hendry, I. A., Stöckel, K., Thoenen, H., and Iversen, L. L. 1974b. The retrograde axonal transport of nerve growth factor. Brain Res. 68:103–121.

Herbert, E., Comb, M., Rosen, H., and Martens, G. 1984. Expression of opioid peptide genes in different species. In Cellular and Molecular Biology ,of Neuronal Development. I. B. Black (ed.), pp. 279–292. Plenum Press, New York.

Hirata, M., and Hayaishi, O. 1967. Adenyl cyclase in brevibacterium liquefaciens. Biochem. Biophys. Acts. 149:1.

Hisada, M. 1957. Membrane resting and action potentials from a protozoan noctituca scintillas. J. Cell Comp. Physiol. 50:57.

Hofstadter, D. R. 1979. Godel, Escher, Bach: An Eternal Golden Braid. Basic Books, New York.

Hokfelt, T., Rehfeld, J. F., Skirboll, L., Ivemark, B., Goldstein, M., and Markey, K. 1980a. Evidence for coexistence of dopamine and CCK in mesolimbic neurones. Nature (Lond.), 285:476–478.

Hokfelt, T. Skirboll, L., Rehfeld, J. F., Goldstein, M., Markey, K., and Dann, O. 1980b. A subpopulation of mesencephalic dopamine neurons projecting to limbic areas contain a cholecystokinin-like peptide: evidence from immunohistochemistry combined with retrograde tracing. Neurosci. 5:2093–2124.

Hokfelt, T., Fuxe, K., and Pernow, V. (eds.). 1986. *Coexistence of Neuronal Messengers: A New Principle in Chemical Transmission*. Elsevier, New York.

Hokfelt, T., Holets, V. R., Staines, W., Meister, B., Melander, T., Schalling, M., Schultzberg, M., Freedman, J., Bjorklund, H., Lars, O., Lindh, B., Elfin, L.-G., Lundberg, J. M., Lindgren, J. A., Samuelsson, B. , Pernow, B., Terenius, L., Post, C., Everitt, B., and Goldstein, M. 1986. Coexistence of neuronal messengers - an overview. In *Progress in Brain Research*, T. Hokfelt, K. Fuxe, and B. Pernow (eds.), vol. 68, pp. 33–70. Elsevier Science Publishers B.V. (Biomedical Division), New York.

Huff, R. M., and Molinoff, P. B. 1982. Quantitative determination of dopamine receptor subtypes not linked to activation of adenylate cyclase in rat striatum. Proc. Natl. Acad. Sci. USA 79:7561–7565.

Hughes, J., Smith, T. W., Kosterlitz, H. W., Fothergill, L. A., Morgan, B. A., and Morris, H. R. 1975. Identification of two related pentapeptides from the brain with potent opiate agonist activity. Nature 258:577–579.

Iversen, L. L. 1967, *The Uptake and Storage of Noradrenaline in Sympathetic Nerves*. Cambridge University Press, London.

Janakidevi, L., Dewey, V. C., and Kidder, 1966. The biosynthesis of catecholamines and the biosynthesis of catecholamines in two genera of protozoa. J. Biol. Chem. 241:2576.

Johnson, E. M., Jr., Andres, R. Y., and Bradshaw, R. A. 1978. Characterization of the retrograde transport of nerve growth factor (NGF) using high specific activity ([125I])NGF. Brain Res. 150:319–331.

Kaas, J. H., Merzenich, M. M., and Killackey, H. P. 1983. The reorganization of somatosensory cortex following peripheral nerve damage in adult and developing mammals. Ann. Review Neurosci. 6:325–356.

Kakidani, H., Furutani, Y., Takahashi, H., Noda, M., Morimoto, Y., Hirose, T., Asai, M., Inayama, S., Nakanishi, S., and Numa, S. 1982. Cloning and sequence analysis of cDNA for porcine beta-neoendorphin/dynorphin precursor. Nature 298:245–249.

Kandel, E. R. 1976. *Cellular Basis of Behavior*. W. H. Freeman and Company, San Francisco.

Kandel, E. R., and Schwartz, J. H. 1982. Molecular biology of learning: Modulation of transmitter release. Science 218:433–443.

Kangawa, K., Minamino, N., Chino, N., Sakakibara, S., and Matsuo, H. 1981. The complete amino acid sequence of alpha-neo-endorphin. Biochem. Biophys. Res. Commun. 99:871–878.

Katz, D. 1969. *The Release of Neural Transmitter Substances*. Schillington Lectures 10. Liverpool University Press, Liverpool.

Kawamura, K., and Chiba, M. 1979. Cortical neurons projecting to the pontine nuclei in the cat. On experimental study with the horseradish peroxidase technique. Exp. Br. Res. 35:269–285.

Keirns, J. J., Carritt, B., Freeman, J., Eisenstadt, J. M., and Bitensky, M. W. 1973. Adenosine 3', 5' cyclic monophosphate in Euglena Gracilis. Life Sci. 13:287.

Kessler, J. A., and Black, I. B. 1979. The role of axonal transport in the regulation of enzyme activity in sympathetic ganglia of adult rats. Brain Res. 171:415–424.

Kessler, J. A., and Black, I. B. 1980. Nerve growth factor stimulates the development of substance P in sensory ganglia. Proc. Natl. Acad. Sci. USA 77:649–652.

Kessler, J. A., and Black, I. B. 1982. Regulation of substance P in adult rat sympathetic ganglia. Brain Res. 234:182–187.

Kessler, J. A., Adler, J. E., and Black, I. B. 1983a. Substance P and somatostatin regulate sympathetic noradrenergic function. Science 221:1059–1061.

Kessler, J. A., Adler, J. E., Bohn, M. C., and Black, I. B. 1981. Substance P in principal sympathetic neurons: Regulation by impulse activity Science 214:335–336.

Kessler, J. A., Bell, W. O., and Black, I. B. 1983b. Interactions between the sympathetic and sensory innervation of the iris. J. Neurosci. 3:1301–1307.

Kimura, S., Lewis, R. V., Stern, A. S., Rosier, J., Stein, S., and Udenfriend, S. 1980. Probable precursors of [Leu] and [Met]enkephalin in adrenal medulla: Peptides of 3–5 kilodaltons. Proc. Natl. Acad. Sci. USA 77:1681–1685.

Korsching, S., and Thoenen, H. 1983. Nerve growth factor in sympathetic ganglia and corresponding target organs of the rat: Correlation with density of sympathetic innervation. Proc. Natl. Acad. Sci. USA 80:3513–3516.

Kosslyn, S. M. 1988. Aspects of a cognitive neuroscience of mental imagery. Science 240:1621–1626.

Korsching, S., Auburger, G., Heumann, R., Scott, J., and Thoenen, H. 1985. Levels of nerve growth factor and its mRNA in the central nervous system of the rat correlate with cholinergic innervation. EMBO J. 4:1389–1393.

Kromer, L. F. 1987. Nerve growth factor treatment after brain injury prevents neuronal death. Science 235:214–216.

Ksir, C. J. 1974. Scopolamine effects on two-trial, delayed-response performance in the rat. Psychopharmacologia 34:127–134.

Kuffler, S. W., Nichols, J. G., and Martin, R. A. 1984. From Neuron to Brain. 2d ed. Sinauer Associates, Sunderland, MA.

Kuhar, J. J. 1976. The anatomy of cholinergic neurons. In Biology of Cholinergic Function, A. M. Goldberg and I. Hanin (eds.), p. 3. Raven, New York.

LaGamma, E. F., and Black, I. B. 1989. Transcriptional control of adrenal catecholamine and opiate peptide transmitter genes. Molec. Br. Res. 5:17–22.

LaGamma, E. F., Adler, J. E., and Black, I. B. 1984. Impulse activity differentially regulates leu-enkephalin and catecholamine characters in the adrenal medulla. Science 224:1102–1104.

LaGamma, E. F., White, J. D., Adler, J. E., Krause, J. E., McKelvy, J. F., and Black, I. B. 1985. Depolarization regulates adrenal preproenkephalin mRNA. Proc. Natl. Acad. Sci. USA 82:8252–8255.

Langer, S. Z. 1974. Presynaptic regulation of catecholamine release. Biochem. Pharmacol. 23:1793–1800.

Large, T. H., Bodary, S. C., Clegg, D. O., and Weskamp, G., Otten, U., and Reichardt, L. F. 1986. Nerve growth factor gene expression in the developing rat brain. Science 234:352–355.

Leibrock, J., Lottspeich, F., Hohn, A., Hofer, M., Hengerer, B., Masiakowski, P., Thoenen, H., and Barde, Y.-A. 1989. Molecular cloning and expression of brain-derived neurotrophic factor. Nature 341:149–152.

Lentz, T. L. 1965a. Fine structural changes in the nervous system of the regenerating hydra. J. Exp. Zool. 159:181.

Lentz, T. L. 1965b. Hydra: Induction of supernumerary heads by isolated neurosecretory granules. Science 150:633.

Lentz, T. L. 1966. Histochemical localization of neurohumors in a sponge. J. Exp. Zool. 162:171.

Lentz, T. L. 1968. Primitive Nervous Systems. Yale Univ. Press, New Haven.

Lentz, T. L., and Barnett, R. J. 1963. The role of the nervous system in regenerating hydras: The effect of neuropharmacological agents. J. Exp. Zool. 154:305.

Lerner, P., Nose, P., Gordon, E. K., and Lovenberg, W. 1977. Haloperidol: Effect of long-term treatment on rat striatal dopamine synthesis and turnover. Science 197:181–182.

Lesh, G. E., and Burnett, A. L. 1966. An analysis of the chemical control of paralized form in hydra. J. Exp. Zool. *163*:55.

Levi-Montalcini, R., and Angeletti, P.U. 1968. Nerve growth factor. Physiol. Rev. *48*:534–569.

Levitt, M., Spector, S., Sjoerdsma, A., and Udenfriend, S. 1965. Elucidation of the rate-limiting step in norepinephrine biosynthesis in the perfused guinea pig heart. J. Pharmacol. Exp. Ther. *148*:1–8.

Lewin, B. 1983. *Genes*. John Wiley & Sons, New York.

Livett, B. G., Dean, D. M., Whelan, L.G., Udenfriend, S., and Rossier, J. 1981. Co-release of enkephalin and catecholamines from cultured adrenal chromaffin cells. Nature (Lond.) *289*:317–319.

Livingstone, M., and Hubel, D. 1988. Segregation of form, color, movement, and depth: Anatomy, physiology, and perception. Science *240*:740–749.

Lu, B., Buck, C. R., Dreyfus, C. F., and Black, I. B. 1989. Expression of NGF in the developing brain: Evidence for local delivery and action of NGF. Exper. Neurol. *104*:191–199.

Lu, B., Yokoyama, M., Dreyfus, C. F., and Black, I. B. 1989. Expression of the NGF gene in dissociated, cultured rat hippocampal cells. Soc. Neurosci. Abstr. *15*:953.

Lundberg, J. M., and Hökfelt, T. 1986. Multiple co-existence of peptides and classical transmitters in peripheral autonomic and sensory neurons—Functional and pharmacological implications. In *Progress in Brain Research*, T. Hökfelt, K. Fuxe and B. Pernow (eds.), vol. 68, pp. 241–262. Elsevier Science Publishers B.V. (Biomedical Division), New York.

Lynch, G. 1986. *Synapses, Circuits, and the Beginnings of Memory*. MIT Press, Cambridge, MA.

Lynch, G., and Baudry, M. 1984. The biochemistry of memory: A new and specific hypothesis. Science *224*:1057–1063.

Macagno, E. R., Lopresti, R. V., and Levinthal, C. 1973. Structure and development of neuronal connections in isogenic organisms: Variations and similarities in the optic system of daphnia magna Proc. Natl. Acad. Sci. USA *70*:57–61.

McClintock, M. K. 1971. Menstrual synchrony and suppression. Nature (Lond.) *229*:244–245.

McClintock, M. K. 1978. Estrous synchrony and its mediation by airborne chemical communication (Rattus norvegicus). Horm. Behav. *10*:264–276.

McClintock, M. K. 1981. Social control of the ovarian cycle and the function of estrus synchrony. Am. Zool. *21*:243–256.

McGaugh, J. L. 1985. *Memory Systems in the Brain: Animal and Human Cognitive Processes*. Edited by M. Weinberger, James L. McGaugh, and Gary Lynch. Guilford Press, New York.

McGeer, E. G., Fibiger, H. C., McGeer, P. L., and Brooke, S. 1973. Temporal changes in amine synthesizing enzymes of rat extrapyramidal structures after hemitransections or 6-hydroxydopamine administration. Brain Res. *52*:289–300.

McHugh, P. 1982. The Concept of Disease in Psychiatry. In *Cecil Textbook of Medicine*, J. B. Wyngaarden and L. H. Smith, Jr. (eds.), 7th ed., pp. 1983–1984. W. B. Saunders Company, Philadelphia.

Mahon, A. C., Nambu, J. R., Taussig, R., Shyamala, M., Roach, A., and Scheller, R. H. 1985. Structure and expression of the egg-laying hormone gene family in aplysia. J. Neurosci. *5*:1872–1880.

Mallet, J., Faucon Biguet, N., Buda, M., Lamouroux, A., and Samolyk, D. 1983. Detection and regulation of the tyrosine hydroxylase mRNA levels in rat adrenal medulla and brain tissues. Cold Spring Harbor Symp. Quant. Biol. *48*:305–308.

Manthorpe, M., and Varon, S. 1985. Regulation of neuronal survival and neuritic growth in the avian ciliary ganglion by trophic factors. In *Growth and Maturation Factors*, G. Guroff (ed.), vol. 3, pp. 77–117. John Wiley & Sons, New York.

Manthorpe, M., Skaper, S., Williams, L. R., and Varon, S. 1986. Purification of adult rat sciatic nerve ciliary neuronotrophic factor. Brain Res. 367:282–286.

Martinez, H. J., Dreyfus, C. F., Jonakait, G. M., and Black, I. B. 1985. Nerve growth factor promotes cholinergic development in brain striatal cultures. Proc. Natl. Acad. Sci. USA 82:7777–7781.

Martinez, H. J., Dreyfus, C. F., Jonakait, G. M., and Black, I. B. 1987. Nerve growth factor selectively increases cholinergic markers but not neuropeptides in rat basal forebrain in culture. Brain Res. 412:295—301.

Mason, S. T., and Fibiger, H. C. 1979. I. Anxiety: The locus coeruleus disconnection. Current Concepts in Life Sciences 25:2141–2147.

Mayr, E. 1981. Biological classification: toward a synthesis of opposing methodologies. Science 214:510.

Melander, T., Hokfelt, T., Rokaeus, A., Cuello, A. C., Oertel, W. H., Verhofstad, A., and Goldstein, M. 1986. Coexistence of galanin-like immunoreactivity with cate-cholamines 5-hydroxytryptamine, GABA and neuropeptides in the rat CNS. J. Neurosci. 6:3640–3654.

Mellander, S. 1960. Comparative studies on the adrenergic neurohormonal control of resistance and capacitance blood vessels in the cat. Acta Physiol. Scand. 50·suppl. 176.

Mesulam, M. M 1989. Behavioral neuroanatomy of cholinergic innervation in the primate cerebral cortex. Experientia-Suppl. 57:1–11.

Mesulam, M. M., and Geula, C. 1988. Nucleus basalis (Ch4) and cortical cholinergic innervation in the human brain: observations based on the distribution of acetyl-cholinesterase and choline acetyltransferase. J. Comp. Neurol. 275:216–240.

Mesulam, M. M., Mufson, E. J., Levey, A. I., and Wainer, B. H. 1984. Atlas of cholinergic neurons in the forebrain and upper brainstem of the macaque based on monoclonal choline acetyltransferase immunohistochemistry and acetylcholinesterase histo-chemistry. Neurosc. 12:669–686.

Mesulam, M. M., Mufson, E. J., and Wainer, B. H. 1986. Three dimensional represen-tation and cortical projection topography of the nucleus basalis (Ch4) in the ma-caque: concurrent demonstration of choline acetyltransferase and retrograde transport with a stabilized tetramethylbenzidine method for horseradish peroxi-dase. Brain Res. 367:301–308.

Meyer, D. K., and Krause, J. 1983. Dopamine modulates cholecystokinin release in neostriatum. Nature (Lond.) 301:338–340.

Meyers, B., and Domino, E. F. 1964. The effect of cholinergic blocking drugs on spon-taneous alternation in rats. Arch. Int. Pharmacodyn. 150:3–4.

Milner, B. 1959. The memory defect in bilateral hippocampal lesions. Psych. Res. Reports 11:43–58.

Milner, B. 1962. Les troubles de la mémoire accompagnant des lesions hippocampiques bilaterales. Physiologie de l'Hippocampe. 107:257–272.

Milner, B. 1970. Memory and the medial temporal regions of the brain. In *Biology of Memory*. K. H. Pribram and D. E. Broadbent (eds.), pp. 29–50. Academic Press, New York.

Milner, B., and Petrides, M. 1984. Behavioural effects of frontal-lobe lesions in man. TINS 7:403–407.

Minneman, K. P., Pittman, R. B., and Molinoff, P. B. 1981. α-adrenergic receptor subtypes: properties, distribution and regulation. Ann. Rev. Neurosci. 4:419–461.

Mishkin, M. 1982. A memory system in the monkey. Phil. Trans. R. Soc. Lond. B 298:85–95.

Mishkin, M., Malamut, B., and Bachevalier, J. 1984. Memories and habits: Two neural systems. In *The Neurobiology of Learning and Memory,* J. L. McGaugh, G. Lynch, and N. M. Weinberger (eds.), pp. 65–77. Guilford Press, New York.

Mitchell, R., and Fleetwood-Walker, S. 1981. Substance P, but not TRH, modulates the 5-HT autoreceptor in ventral lumbar spinal cord. Europ. J. Pharmacol. 76:119–120.

Mizuno, K., Minamino, N., Kangawa, K., and Matsuo, H. 1980. A new family of endogenous "big" [Met]enkephalins from bovine adrenal medulla: Purification and structure of docosa-(BAM22P) and eicosapeptide (BAM) with very potent opiate activity. Biochem. Biophys. Res. Commun. 97:1283–1290.

Mobley, W. C., Rutkowski, J. L., Tennekoon, G. I., Buchanan, K., and Johnston, M. V. 1985. Choline acetyltransferase activity in striatum of neonatal rats increased by nerve growth factor. Science 229:284–287.

Mobley, W. C., Rutkowski, J. L., Tennekoon, G. I., Gemski, J., Buchanan, K., and Johnston, M. V. 1986. Nerve growth factor increases choline acetyltransferase activity in developing basal forebrain neurons. Mol. Brain Res. 1:53–62.

Molinoff, P. B., and Axelrod, J. 1971. Biochemistry of catecholamines. Ann. Rev. Biochem. 49:465–500.

Moore, R. Y., and Bloom, F. E. 1978. Central catecholamine neuron systems: Anatomy and physiology of the dopamine systems. Ann. Rev. Neurosci. 2:129–169.

Moore, R. Y., and Bloom, F. E. 1979. Central catecholamine neuron systems: anatomy and physiology of the norepinephrine and epinephrine systems. Ann. Rev. Neurosci. 2:113–168.

Morrison, J. R. 1973. Catatonia, retarded and excited types. Arch. Gen. Psych. 28:39.

Morrison, R. S., Kornblum, H. I., Leslie, F. M., and Bradshaw, R. A. 1987. Trophic stimulation of cultured neurons from neonatal fat brain by epidermal growth factor. Science 238:72–75.

Morrison, R. S., Sharma, A., DeVellis, J., and Bradshaw, R. A. 1986. Basic fibroblast growth factor supports the survival of cerebral cortical neurons in primary cultures. Proc. Natl. Acad. Sci. USA 83:7537–7541.

Mudge, A. W. 1989. Neuropeptides find a role? Nature 339:663.

Mueller, R. A., Thoenen, H., and Axelrod, J. 1969. Increase in tyrosine hydroxylase activity after reserpine administration. J. Pharmac. Exp. Ther. 169:74–79.

Murrin, L. C., Morgenroth, V. H. III, and Roth, R. H. 1976. Dopaminergic neurons: Effects of electrical stimulation on tyrosine hydroxylase. Molec. Pharmcol. 2:1070–1081.

Nestler, E. J. and Greengard, P. 1984. *Protein Phosphorylation in the Nervous System.* Wiley, New York.

Newell, A. 1980. Physical symbol systems. Cognitive Science 4:135–183.

Nicoll, R. A. 1988. The coupling of neurotransmitter receptors to ion channels in the brain. Science 241:545–52.

Nicoll, R. A., Kauer, J. A., and Malenka, R. C. 1988. The current excitement in long-term potentiation. Neuron. 1(2):97–103.

Noda, M., Furutani, Y., Takahashi, H., Toyosato, M., Hirose, T., Inayama, S., Nakanishi, S., and Numa, S. 1982a. Cloning and sequence analysis of cDNA for bovine adrenal preproenkephalin. Nature 295:202–206.

Noda, M., Teranishi, Y., Takahashi, H., Toyosato, M., Notake, M., Nakanishi, S., and Numa, S. 1982b. Isolation and structural organization of the human preproenkephalin gene. Nature 297:431.

Nygren, L. G., and Olson, L. 1977. A new major projection from locus coeruleus: The main source of noradrenergic nerve terminals in the ventral and dorsal columns of the cord. Brain Res. *132*:85–94.

Okaichi, H., and Jarrard, L. E. 1982. Scopolamine impairs performance of a place and cue task in rats. Behav. and Neural Biol. *35*:319–325.

O'Keefe, J., and Nadel, L. 1978. *The Hippocampus as a Cognitive Map*. Oxford University Press, London.

Olton, D. S. 1989. Mnemonic functions of the hippocampus: Single unit analyses in rats. In *The Hippocampus—New Vistas*, pp. 411–424. Alan R. Liss, New York.

Olton, D. S., Becker, J. T., and Handelmann, G. E. 1979. Hippocampus, space and memory. In *The Behavioral and Brain Sciences*, vol. 2, pp. 313–365. Cambridge University Press, Cambridge.

Orgel, L. E. 1973. *The Origins of Life: Molecules and Natural Selection*. John Wiley & Sons, New York.

Parker, G. H. 1919. *The Elementary Nervous System*. Lippincott, Philadelphia.

Patterson, P. H. 1978. Environmental determination of autonomic neurotransmitter functions. Ann. Rev. Neurosci. *1*:1–17.

Piattelli-Palmarini, M., ed. 1979. *Language and Learning*. Harvard University Press, Cambridge, MA.

Pincus, D. W., DiCicco-Bloom, E., and Black, I. B. 1990. Vasoactive intestinal peptide regulates mitosis, differentiation and survival of cultured sympathetic neuroblasts. Nature *343*:564–567.

Purves, D. 1988. *Body and Brain: A Trophic Theory of Neural Connections*. Harvard University Press, Cambridge, MA.

Pylyshyn, Z. 1980. Computation and cognition: Issues in the foundations of cognitive science. Behav. Brain Sci. *3*:111–132.

Redmond, D. E., Jr., and Huang, Y. H. 1979. II. New evidence for a locus coeruleus-norepinephrine connection with anxiety. Current Concepts in Life Sciences *25*:2149–2162.

Redmond, D. E., Huang, Y. H., Snyder, D. R., and Maas, J. W. 1976. Behavioral effects of stimulation of the nucleus locus coeruleus in the stump-tailed monkey macaca arctoides. Brain Res. *116*:502–510.

Roach, A., Adler, J. E., and Black, I. B. 1987. Depolarizing influences regulate preprotachykinin mRNA in sympathetic neurons. Proc. Natl. Acad. Sci. USA *84*:5078–5081.

Rosensweig, Z., and Kindler, S. H. 1972. Epinephrine and serotonin activation of adrenyl cyclase from tetrahymena pyriformis. FEBS Lett. *25*:221.

Rumelhart, D. E., and McClelland, J. L. 1986. *Parallel Distributed Processing*. MIT Press, Cambridge, MA.

Rutishauser, U., and Jessell, T. 1988. Cell adhesion molecules in vertebrate neural development. Physiol. Rev. *68*:819–857.

Rye, D. B., Wainer, B. H., Mesulam, M. M., Mufson, B. J., and Saper, C. B. 1984. Cortical projections arising from the basal forebrain: A study of cholinergic and noncholinergic components employing combined retrograde tracing and immunohistochemical localization of choline acetyltransferase. Neurosci. *13*:627–643.

Sabban, E., Goldstein, M., Bohn, M. C., and Black, I. B. 1982. Development of the adrenergic phenotype: Increase in adrenal messenger RNA coding for phenylethanolamine-N-methyltransferase. Proc. Natl. Acad. Sci. USA *79*:4823–4827.

Schaller, H. C. 1983. Hormonal regulation of regeneration in hydra. In *Current Methods in Cellular Neurobiology*, J. L. Barker and J. F. McKelvy (eds.), vol. 4, pp. 1–14. John Wiley & Sons, New York.

Scheller, R. H., Jackson, J. F., McAllister, L. B., Rothman, B. S., Mayer, E., and Axel, R. 1983a. A single gene encodes multiple neuropeptides mediating a stereotyped behavior. Cell 32:7–22.

Scheller, R. H., Jackson, J. F., McAllister, L. B., Schwartz, J. H., Kandel, E. R., and Axel, R. 1982. A family of genes that codes for ELH, a neuropeptide eliciting a stereotyped pattern of behavior in aplysia. Cell 28:707–719.

Scheller, R. H., Rothman, B. S., and Mayeri, E. 1983b. A single gene encodes multiple peptide-transmitter candidates involved in a stereotyped behavior. TINS. 6:340–345.

Schildkraut, J. J., and Kety, S. S. 1967. Biogenic amines and emotion. Science 156:21–30.

Schultzberg, M., Foster, G. A., Gage, F. H., Björklund, A., and Hökfelt, T. 1986. Coexistence during ontogeny and transplantation. In Progress in Brain Research, T. Hokfelt, K. Fuxe, and B. Pernow (eds.), vol. 68, pp. 129–145. Elsevier Science Publishers B.V. (Biomedical Division), New York.

Schwab, M. E., Otten, U., Agid, Y., and Thoenen, H. 1979. Nerve growth factor (NGF) in the rat CNS: Absence of specific retrograde axonal transport and tyrosine hydroxylase induction in locus coeruleus and substantia nigra. Brain Res. 168:473–483.

Shelton, D. L., and Reichardt, L. F. 1984. Expression of the β-nerve growth factor gene correlates with the density of sympathetic innervation in effector organs. Proc. Natl. Acad. Sci. USA 81:7951–7955.

Shelton, D. L., and Reichardt, L. F. 1986. Studies on the expression of the β-nerve growth factor (NGF) gene in the central nervous system: Level and regional distribution of NGF mRNA suggest that NGF functions as a trophic factor for several distinct populations of neurons. Proc. Natl. Acad. Sci. USA 83:2714–2718.

Shepherd, G. M. 1986. Apical dentritic binds of cortical pyramidal cells: Remarks on their possible roles in higher brain functions, including memory. In Synapses, Circuits, and the Beginnings of Memory, G. Lynch, pp. 85–98. MIT Press, Cambridge, MA.

Shuttleworth, E. C., and Wise, G. R. 1973. Transient global amnesia due to arterial embolism. Arch. Neurol. 29:340–342.

Siekevitz, P. 1985. The postsynaptic density: A possible role in long-lasting effects in the central nervous system. Proc. Natl. Acad. Sci. USA. 82:3494–3498.

Skirboll, L. R., Crawley, J. N., and Hommer, D. W. 1986. Functional studies of cholecystokinin-dopamine coexistence: electrophysiology and behavior. In Progress in Brain Research. T. Hokfelt, K. Fuxe, and B. Pernow, (eds.), vol. 68, pp. 357–367. Elsevier Science Publishers B.V. (Biomedical Division), New York.

Smith, A. B. III., Belcher, A. M., Epple, G., Jurs, P. C., and Lavine, B. 1985. Computerized pattern rcognition: A new technique for the analysis of chemical communication. Science 228:175–177.

Smylie, C. S., Baynes, K. M., Hirst, W., and McCleary, C. 1984. Profiles of right hemisphere language and speech following brain bisection. Brain Lang. 22:206.

Snowdon, C. T. 1983. Ethology, comparative psychology, and animal behavior. Ann. Rev. Psychol. 34:63–94.

Squire, L. R. 1986. Mechanisms of memory. Science 232:1612–1619.

Stachowiak, M., Sebbane, R., Stricker, E. M., Zigmond, M. J., and Kaplan, B. B. 1985. Effect of chronic cold exposure on tyrosine hydroxylase mRNA in rat adrenal gland. Brain Res. 359:356–360.

Stjarne, L., and Lundberg, J. M. 1986. On the possible roles of noradrenaline, adenosine 5'-triphosphate and neuropeptide Y as sympathetic cotransmitters in the mouse vas deferens. In Progress in Brain Research. T. Hokfelt, K. Fuxe, and B. Pernow (eds.), vol. 68, pp. 263–278. Elsevier Science Publishers B.V. (Biomedical Division), New York.

Stockel, K., Schwab, M., and Thoenen, H. 1975a. Comparison between the retrograde axonal transport of nerve growth factor and tetanus toxin in motor, sensory and adrenergic neurons. Brain Res. 99:1–16.

Stockel, K., Schwab. M., and Thoenen, H. 1975b. Specificity of retrograde transport of nerve growth factor (NGF) in sensory neurons: A biochemical and morphological study. Brain Res. 89:1–14.

Sutter, A., Hosang, M., Vale R. D., and Shooter, E. M. 1984. The interaction of nerve growth factor with it specific receptors. In Cellular and Molecular Biology of Neuronal Development, I. B. Black (ed.). Plenum Press, New York.

Swanson, L., Cowan, W. M., and Jones, T. 1974. An autoradiographic study of the afferent connections of the ventral lateral geniculate nucleus in the albino rat and the cat. J. Comp. Neurol. 156:143–164.

Swanson, L. W., and Hartman, B. K. 1975. The central adrenergic system. An immunofluorescence study of the location of cell bodies and their efferent connections in the rat utilizing dopamine-beta-hydroxylase as a marker. J. Comp. Neurol. 163:467–506.

Swanson, L.W., Sawchenko, P. E., and Lind, R. W. 1986. Regulation of multiple peptides in CRF parvocellular neurosecretory neurons: Implications for the stress response. In Progress in Brain Research, T. Hokfelt, K. Fuxe, and B. Pernow (eds.), vol. 68, pp. 169–190. Elsevier Science Publishers B.V. (Biomedical Division), New York.

Sy, J., and Richter, D. 1972. Content of cyclic 3', 5'-adenosine. Biochem. 11:2788.

Thierry, A. M., Tassin, J. P., and Glowinski, J. 1984. Functional properties: Introductory remarks. In Monoamine Innervation of Cerebral Cortex, L. Descarries and H. H. Jasper (eds.), pp. 229–232. Alan R. Liss, New York.

Thoenen, H., Angeletti, P. U., Levi-Montalcini, R., and Kettler, R. 1971. Selective induction by nerve growth factor of tyrosine hydroxylase and dopamine-β hydroxylase in rat superior cervical ganglia. Proc. Natl. Acad. Sci. USA 68:1598–1602.

Thoenen, H., Mueller, R. A., and Axelrod, J. 1969. Transsynaptic induction of adrenal tyrosine hydroxylase. J. Pharmac. Exp. Ther. 169:249–254.

Thoenen, H., Mueller, R. A. and Axelrod, J. 1970. Phase difference in the induction of tyrosine hydroxylase in cell body and nerve terminals of sympathetic neurons. Proc Natl. Acad. Sci. USA 65:58–62.

Thompson, R. F. 1986. The neurobiology of learning and memory. Science 233:941–947.

Tomkins, G. M. 1975. Metabolic Code—Biological symbolism and the origin of intercellular communications is discussed. Science 189:760.

Truex, R. C. 1959. Strong and Elwyn's Human Neuroanatomy, 4th ed. Williams & Wilkins, Baltimore, MD.

Varon, S., Manthorpe, M., and Adler, R. 1979. Cholinergic neuronotrophic factors. I. Survival neurite outgrowth and choline acetyltransferase activity in monolayer cultures from chick embryo ciliar ganglia. Brain Res. 173:29–45.

Viveros, O. H., Diliberto, E. J., Hazum, E., and Chang, K.-J. 1979. Opiate-like materials in the adrenal medulla: evidence for storage and secretion with catecholamines. Molec. Pharmacol. 16:1101–1108.

Walicke, P. 1988. Basic and acidic fibroblast growth factors have trophic effects on neurons from multiple CNS regions. J. Neurosci. 8:2618–2627.

Walicke, P., and Baird, A. 1988. Neurotrophic effects of basic acidic fibroblast growth factors are not mediated through glial cells. Dev. Brain Res. 40:71–79.

Walicke, P., Cowan, W. M., Ueno, N., Baird, A., and Guillemin, R. 1986. Fibroblast growth factor promotes survival of dissociated hippocampal neurons and enhances neurite extension. Proc. Natl. Acad. Sci. USA 73:4210–4114.

Walker, J. M., Akil, H., and Watson, S. J. 1980a. Evidence for homologous actions of proopiocortin products. Science 210:1247–1249.

Walker, J. M., Katz, R. J., and Akil, H. 1980b. Behavioral effects of dynorphin-(1–13) in the mouse and rat: Initial observations. Peptides 1:341–345.

Waymire, J. C., Johnston, J. P., Hummer-Lickteig, K., Lloyd, A., Vigny, A., and Craviso, G. L. 1988. Phosphorylation of bovine adrenal chromaffin cell tyrosine hydroxylase: Temporal correlation of acetylcholines effect on sight phosphorylation, enzyme activation and catecholamine synthesis. J. Biol. Chem. 263:12439–47.

Welch, G. R. 1987. The living cell as an ecosystem: Hierarchical analogy and symmetry. TREE 2:305–309.

Westlind, A., Grynfarb, M., Hedlund, B., Bartfai, T., and Fuxe, K. 1981. Muscarinic supersensitivity induced by septal lesion or chronic atropine treatment. Brain Res. 225:131–141.

Whitehouse, P. J., Price, D. L., Clark, A. W., Coyle, J. T., and DeLong, M. R. 1981. Alzheimer's disease: Evidence for selective loss of cholinergic neurons in the nucleus basalis. Ann. Neurol. 10:122.

Whitehouse, P. J., Price, D. L., Struble, R. G., Clark, A. W., Coyle, J. T., and DeLong, M. R. 1982. Alzheimer's disease and senile dementia: Loss of neurons in the basal forebrain. Science 215:1237.

Whittaker, R. W. 1969. New concepts of kingdoms of organisms. Evolutionary relations are better represented by new classifications than by the traditional two kingdoms. Science 163:150.

Whittemore, S. R., and Seiger, A. 1987. The expression, localization and functional significance of β-nerve growth factor in the central nervous system. Brain Res. Rev. 12:439–464.

Weiner, S. I., Paul, C. A., and Eichenbaum, H. 1989. Spatial and behavioral correlates of hippocampal neuronal activity. J. Neurosci. 9:2737–2763.

Williams, L. R., Varon, S., Peterson, G. M., Wictorin, K., Fischer, W., Björklund, A., and Gage, F. H. 1986. Continuous infusion of nerve growth factor prevents basal forebrain neuronal death after fimbria fornix transection. Proc. Natl. Acad. Sci. USA 83:9231–9235.

Wilson, S. P., Chang, K.-J., and Viveros, O. H. 1982. Proportional secretion of opioid peptides and catecholamines from adrenal chromaffin cells in culture. J. Neurosci. 2:1150–1156.

Wirsching, B. A., Beninger, R. J., Jhamandas, K., Boegman, R. J., and El-Defrawy, S. R. 1984. Differential effects of scopolamine on working and reference memory of rats in the radial maze. Pharmacol. Biochem. Behav. 20:659–662.

Wu, K., and Black, I. B. 1989. Regulation of synaptic molecular architecture in a rat sympathetic ganglion and hippocampus. J. Cognitive Neurosci. 1:194–200.

Yokota, T., and Gots, J. S. 1970. Requirement of adenosine 3′, 5′-cyclic phosphate for flagella formation in escherichia coli and salmanella typhimurium. J. Bacteriol. 103:513.

Zaidel, E. 1983. Disconnection syndrome as a model for laterality effects in the normal brain. In Cerebral Hemisphere Asymmetry: Method, Theory and Application. J. B. Helige (ed.), pp. 95–151. Praeger, New York.

Zigmond, R. E. 1979. Tyrosine hydroxylase activity in noradrenergic neurons of the locus coeruleus after reserpine administration: sequential increase in cell bodies and nerve terminals. J. Neurochem. 32:23–29.

Zigmond, R. E. 1980a. Preganglionic nerve stimulation increases the amount of tyrosine hydroxylase in the rat superior cervical ganglion. Neurosci. Lett. 20:61–65.

Zigmond, R. E. 1980b. The long-term regulation of ganglionic tyrosine hydroxylase by preganglionic nerve activity. Fed. Proc. 39:3003–3008.

Zigmond, R. E., and Chalazonitis, A. 1979. Long-term effects of preganglionic nerve stimulation on tyrosine hydroxylase activity in the rat superior cervical ganglion. Brain Res. 164:137–152.

Zigmond, R. E., and Mackay, A. V. P. 1974. Dissociation of stimulatory and synthetic phases in the induction of tyrosine hydroxylase. Nature 247:112–113.

Zigmond, R. E., Schon, F., and Iversen. L. L. 1974. Increased tyrosine hydroxylase activity in the locus coeruleus of rat brain stem after reserpine treatment and cold stress. Brain Res. 70:547–552.

Zigmond, R. E., Schwarzschild, M. A., and Rittenhouse, A. R. 1989. Acute regulation of tyrosine hydroxylase by nerve activity and by neurotransmitters via phosphorylation. Ann. Rev. Neurosci. 12:415–461.

Index